ONE PERSON
AT A TIME

Citizen Advocacy for People
with Disabilities

BY ADAM (A.J.) HILDEBRAND

BROOKLINE BOOKS
Brookline, Massachusetts 02445

ISBN 1-57129-093-1

Library of Congress Cataloging-In-Publication Data

Hildebrand, Adam.
    One person at a time : citizen advocacy for people with disabilities/
by Adam (A.J.) Hildebrand. -- 1st ed.
        p. cm.
    Includes bibliographical references.
    ISBN 1-57129-093-1 (alk. paper)
    1. People with disabilities--Care. 2. People with
disabilities--Services for. I. Title.
    HV1568.H55 2004
    362.4'04525--dc22

2004040710

Printed by
10 9 8 7 6 5 4 3 2 1

For orders:
BROOKLINE BOOKS
P.O. Box 97
Newton, MA 02464

Order toll-free: 1-800-666-BOOK

TABLE OF CONTENTS

FOREWORD

WOLF WOLFENSBERGER

When I first came up with the idea of Citizen Advocacy in a very embryonic form in 1966, the initial response from a lot of people was, "No one will put themselves out voluntarily for a handicapped person to whom they are not related, when they don't have to." Even parents of persons with significant impairments said then that fate had put a very difficult parental role on them that they would not have chosen, and the idea that other people would take on a similar role voluntarily on an unpaid basis was totally unrealistic. But I was convinced that there were people who would — and this book, and the stories related in it — proves that this is so.

However, even though I was convinced that Citizen Advocacy would work, I did not fully anticipate what a dramatic difference it could make in so many lives. Indeed, as you will read in this book, it has built bridges, changed attitudes, opened minds and hearts, changed lives, and even saved many lives — sometimes the same life many times over. I am deeply gratified that this has turned out to be one of the fruits of Citizen Advocacy.

At the same time, my view of what the formal, organized human service system can accomplish has changed over my career. Where once I had high hopes of service reform, and actually witnessed and participated in such dramatic reform, I now see the formal, paid, organized service system to have come to a state of functional collapse, even as it has been getting bigger and bigger every year, and consuming ever more money. The overarching reason for this development is that Western society itself is in a state of collapse, including its capacity to deliver what I call comitous polity, i.e., people being able to live relatively harmoniously together in enough agreement about basic issues so as to be able to make some political system work. This societal collapse is evidenced in increasingly decadent values and lifestyles, the decline of ever more of the kinds of social institutions that can hold a society together, and the crippling formalization that is overtaking much of society. Whatever characterizes a society at large will inevitably express itself in the human service sector, and together with a minority of other people, I believe our formal human service sector in its totality is now wreaking at least as much harm on people as it is benefiting them. However, many people are kept from recognizing this by taking account only of the benefits, in some cases because they are being deceived about the dark side of things.

While it is now dangerous in many ways to become a service client — even for privileged people, to say nothing of already lowly ones — and while individual members of our culture are more and more succumbing to false worldviews and decadence, many can still be challenged to rise to good deeds as private individuals, even when in their roles as members of formal structures, they are inhibited — or even prohibited — from doing so. Thus, more and more, I have come to believe that if anything can be made to work in the lives of devalued people, it is going to be informal, voluntary, freely-given relationships, advocacy, and service. And Citizen Advocacy is one version that this giving can take.

I am very gratified that A.J. Hildebrand, and so many others, have taken the idea of Citizen Advocacy, implemented it, fleshed it out, and here — by writing about it — are passing on to others the lessons of what it can do and what it can teach. The idea of Citizen Advocacy has by now had a positive impact in the lives of many thousands of people. While there is not much in the world of human service about which I am hopeful, I do believe that there will always be individuals who will strive to function as moral actors, and that some people will be more likely to function as such if there is someone who challenges them to do so, as Citizen Advocacy offices are designed to do and are doing.

Wolf Wolfensberger is a Professor in the School of Education at Syracuse University, where he also directs the Training Institute for Human Service Planning, Leadership and Change Agentry.

DAVID B. SCHWARTZ

When I first met Adam (A.J.) Hildebrand, he had just been fired for doing the right thing. This is the kind of clarifying experience that can propel a certain kind of person to depart from ordinary paths and to establish that most difficult of human services: a Citizen Advocacy office. It turned out that A.J. was such a person.

Citizen Advocacy attempts to respond to living in the modern world by the radical act of taking seriously the story of the Good Samaritan — and even pre-Christian traditions of offering hospitality to strangers in one's midst. In a world in which professionals spend lifetimes inventing and managing more complex systems to serve marginalized and devalued people, the citizen advocate's unschooled attempt to lift one stranger from a ditch can be greeted with incredulity, if not hostility.

Citizen Advocacy coordinators face not only external hazards, including a consequent scarcity of funding and the loneliness that can come from treading a path that few understand. They additionally face the temptations of egotism and self-defeating fundamentalism that lie in wait for those who consider themselves special in combating dark forces of oppression.

If one can tread this narrow path successfully, one can encounter the most magic of moments. When a Citizen Advocacy coordinator carefully introduces an isolated person to a potential advocate and the relationship "takes," he or she can watch two mysterious destinies begin to intertwine as each glimpses the true face of the other. Such "askers" catalyze one of the most beautiful events in life: that of seeing someone invite a stranger across the threshold into their heart. Nothing is the same after this.

This collection of stories and commentary is the work of one of the most serious and successful Citizen Advocacy coordinators I have known. It was A.J. and his partner Denise Shaw's work alone, sometimes, that kept my hope in Citizen Advocacy alive. A.J. has done Citizen Advocacy, he has made it work, and he has changed the life-stories of many. He shares his considerable knowledge of this rare art here. In this book one sees why Citizen Advocacy is worth doing.

David B. Schwartz is the author of CROSSING THE RIVER: CREATING A CONCEPTUAL REVOLUTION IN COMMUNITY AND DISABILITY, *and* WHO CARES? REDISCOVERING COMMUNITY. *He is also a former executive director of the Developmental Disabilities Council of Pennsylvania.*

PREFACE

_____

TOM KOHLER

As you read Adam (A.J.) Hildebrand's book, many of you will recognize the journey. This book is about A.J.'s personal journey of trying to understand what is worth doing in the world. It is about the vehicle he used to answer that question for 16 years, and it is about the long journey toward more thoughtful, welcoming and just communities, communities characterized by more respectful and responsible relationships between individual people.

A.J. could have had a career. He was in the right place at the right time. He was working in Pennsylvania, a state that led the fight for more humane services for people with mental retardation in the 1970s. He was working in the late 1970s and early 1980s when legal opinion and idealism, mixed with new federal and state money, was spawning services for people with mental retardation outside of the institutions. A.J. could have parlayed his job in a residential service agency into a regional position and then a state-level position.

A.J. could have had a career, except for two problems. The first problem was that he became inspired. The second is that he became impatient. A.J. became deeply inspired by the work and words of a man named Dr. Wolf Wolfensberger. He became inspired by a way of learning that brought small groups of strangers together for five days at a time and allowed them to look deeply into the lives of people with disabilities and the services they were expected to use. He became inspired as he saw people like Susan Thomas, Darcy Elks, Guy Caruso, Michael Kendrick, Lou Chapman and John O'Brien become leaders in critiquing the present and carving out new ways to think about people, systems and society.

The second problem keeping A.J. from a career was rightful impatience. The gap between what could be worthwhile and possible — and what state-funded agencies were willing to move toward — grew too quickly for A.J. He tried to stay, to work inside the system, to have a career, but he couldn't. Like many other people in the 1970s and early 1980s, A.J. had to leave his work to find good work.

For 16 years, A.J. chose Dr. Wolfensberger's idea of Citizen Advocacy as the vehicle for doing work that he feels is worthwhile and possible. This book is about what A.J. and many other people involved in Citizen Advocacy have learned over roughly 25 years.

I would encourage you to read this book in the following way: Let the stories be the story. Read one or two of the Citizen Advocacy stories in the book and then read a chapter about the philosophy and implementation of Citizen Advocacy. By moving back and forth from concept to story, story to concept, you get the flavor of how Citizen Advocacy really works. Working from a clear set of principles, the Citizen Advocacy staff invites individual citizens into direct personal relationship with one another. As people in Citizen Advocacy relationships learn from one another, the staff and board members of the Citizen Advocacy program learn more about human nature, personal relationships, the nature of change, and the strengths and weaknesses of the Citizen Advocacy model.

I do not understand everything that A.J. is telling me in this book. Part of A.J.'s Citizen Advocacy journey has taken him to a deeply religious place in his life. The more directly the book moves toward the realm of spiritual faith, the less I understand. I have always appreciated A.J.'s willingness to accept our differences in this way. His confidence in his own faith has not been translated into a need to convert me.

There are also parts of this book that I do not agree with. It does not matter what they are. What matters is that there is enough room under the Citizen Advocacy umbrella for a lot of people to stand. Basic assumptions about how the world works and does not work, specifically the position of people with disabilities in historical and current culture, are important. So is an agreement on the structure of Citizen Advocacy as expressed in its definition and principles, and to a lesser extent, its key operational activities. But beyond that, there should be plenty of room under the umbrella for people to learn and to do the work of Citizen Advocacy.

This book has been wrestled from the experience of one man who chose to follow his heart. This book is about a lot of what you see along the way. A.J. did not see everything on his journey. No one does. That is part of what keeps this idea of Citizen Advocacy alive in the hearts and minds of people who are connected to it, the paid staff who are the inviters, and the people who enter into voluntary personal relationship with one another. You know, because of what you have seen, and because of what you have not seen yet, there is plenty more to do. Here, in *One Person At A Time: Citizen Advocacy for People with Disabilities*, A.J. gives us all a chance to review, reflect, and renew our vision and efforts.

Tom Kohler
Citizen Advocacy Coordinator
Chatham-Savannah Citizen Advocacy
Savannah, Georgia

Mr. Kohler has been the Coordinator of Chatham-Savannah Citizen Advocacy since 1978. He continues to meet and match people, one person at a time.

ACKNOWLEDGMENTS

So many people have been part of the work of One to One: Citizen Advocacy in Beaver County, Pennsylvania, and in my work with Citizen Advocacy programs around the world, I hardly know where to begin. Without Wolf Wolfensberger, there would be no Citizen Advocacy, and I acknowledge Wolf's work as a prime mover in my life and work. Someone has said that Citizen Advocacy opens a window through which one sees realities one would not otherwise see. I am grateful for that window, in spite of the difficult things I have seen in contemplating how human beings devalue and oppress one another. Citizen Advocacy, as this book attests, offers a positive way to respond to these realities, and to bring out and build upon the goodness we can call forth in one another.

That brings me to the next person I want to acknowledge, Denise Shaw. Without Denise, there would be no Citizen Advocacy in Beaver County. If not for her talents and energy, we never would have made it off the ground. During our 16 years of work together, Denise and I often joked that between the two of us, we made one good Citizen Advocacy coordinator. Denise brought out the good in me, and I hope I helped bring out the good in her, as we tried day by day to make a difference in our world in Beaver County through Citizen Advocacy.

Without citizen advocates and without the people who opened themselves up to having citizen advocates, there would be no stories to share, no lessons to learn. Naming all the people who gave of themselves, both as advocates and as people who have had advocates, would take many pages. I invite each citizen advocate whom

I have known, every citizen advocate whom I have not known, and each and every person who has an advocate who may read these pages to feel part and parcel of this book in a way that transcends the boundaries of time and space. This book is about you, and people like you.

Board members, especially those who assumed leadership roles at One to One: Citizen Advocacy, kept the ship afloat, and valiantly steered the course in the midst of many storms. I express my deep gratitude to all board members past and present at One to One: Citizen Advocacy, especially our founding board members and board presidents: Paul Gillespie, Crea Snider, Alice Irvin, Harry Smeltz, Pat Cassino, Barb Langhel, Harriet Kulha, Ross Crow, Dean Byrom, Tim Koch, James Ross, Al Catanzarite, Lynn Jessep, Brian Hayden, Kate Kelley, Julie Peck, Linda Nulph and Mary Krepps. These are people who sometimes laid awake at night both dreaming and worrying about how to sustain the presence of Citizen Advocacy in Beaver County.

I am very grateful to David Schwartz and to the Developmental Disabilities Council of Pennsylvania for the support and opportunity to establish One to One: Citizen Advocacy, and to the many private supporters in Pennsylvania who helped sustain One to One: Citizen Advocacy as an organization. Guy Caruso, the board president of Pennsylvania Citizen Advocacy, was key to bringing the idea of Citizen Advocacy to Pennsylvania in the early days, and along with David Schwartz, helped generate support for Citizen Advocacy on a state level.

I am also deeply indebted to the many people who taught me the art and science of Citizen Advocacy, especially: Tom Kohler, Tom Doody, Barbara Fischer, John Murphy, Kathy Alexander, Sherry Cooke, Andra Frank, Andy Baxter, Cecile Lynes, Julie Clarke, Zana Lutfiyya and Lou Chapman.

Three people who have disabilities have had a most significant impact in my life in terms of how I understand what it means to live with a disability and more importantly, what it means to be human. Denise Aiello taught me more about what it means to live with a disability than any other person. Paul Gillespie taught me, and still teaches me, that he and I are the same at the deepest level of our humanity. Renee Circle, who no longer lives in this world, taught me how to love when everything else has failed, when everything else is lost.

Many people made this book possible. The people who share their stories in this book have consented to allow their light to shine on a hill rather than keeping it under a bushel, and I am so very grateful to them for shedding light on the path for the rest of us. Writing and re-writing their stories line-by-line has been a labor of love. The board and staff of Chatham-Savannah Citizen Advocacy were especially helpful in the writing of this book, and provided me with ample opportunity to listen and learn.

Readers, editors and reviewers of many drafts of the manuscript gave me valuable critique, insights and encouragement to keep going. Marc Tumeinski was particularly helpful in both the early and later stages, and gave invaluable advice on organization of chapters and refining the manuscript. Denise Shaw, Stephen Catanzarite, Jennifer Cullen, Tom Kohler, Susan Thomas and Wolf Wolfensberger gave me key feedback that helped me re-orient and focus the work. Jo Massarelli, Joe Osburn, Jack Yates, Susanne Hartfiel, David Schwartz, Dave Lichius, Deb Geeza, and my daughter Kelly McElravy helped with some finer points of editing. Gene Downs, Rich Wittish, Billy Hughes, and Stephen Catanzarite wrote four short stories about Citizen Advocacy relationships, which appear in the first chapter. Milt Budoff, my editor at Brookline Books, graciously provided valuable critique and encouragement along the way, and took the risk of publishing a first-time author. I am especially indebted to the Scaife Family Foundation, the JM Foundation, and an anonymous foundation, whose financial support made writing this book possible.

My more recent work has been focused on the heightened vulnerability of people with disabilities in medical settings, and so I am indebted to Conrad O'Donnell and the Shriver Clinical Services Corporation for supporting this attempt to share what I have learned from Citizen Advocacy while providing consulting opportunities through which I have deepened my understanding of human vulnerability at the margins of society.

Finally, I dedicate this book to my children, Colleen, Kelly and

Michael. They made sacrifices during my intensive years of Citizen Advocacy work. I hope that this book reveals that their sacrifice of some of my time was worthwhile.

INTRODUCTION

This book is for people who want to change the world — particularly the world for people with disabilities — one person at a time. Real change, the change that matters most, is the change that happens in the hearts and minds of individual people in the context of their everyday lives. This begins with an interior transformation of people who realize that to change the world, they must first change themselves. This book describes how this personal transformation can happen in the context of committed, voluntary relationships between people with and without disabilities.

The primary focus of this book is to encourage personal engagement in the lives of people with disabilities. There are two main reasons why such engagement is important. First, genuine personal alliances between people with and without disabilities can have a powerful, positive impact in the lives of people with disabilities. All the social change efforts in the world make little difference unless individual people with disabilities have people in their lives whom they can count on. Having a place in the world begins with having a place in the hearts and minds of other people.

Secondly, personal engagements in the lives of individual people with disabilities benefit those who do not have disabilities. Meaningful, personal engagement in the life of someone with a disability can change non-disabled people for the better. This change is unique to each person and to each relationship, but looking at the world through the eyes of a person with a disability offers an opportunity to learn about human nature and the world in which we live. A relationship with someone who lives with a disability, as in any human relationship, calls one to look in the mirror and honestly deal with what one sees — both the good and the bad. A relationship with a person with a disability offers important lessons about the value and dignity of every human being, and what it means to live as part of the human community.

Human beings are made to be social, to be a part of something bigger than themselves. People with disabilities usually encounter many significant physical and social barriers to developing such connections with typical people. Disabled and non-disabled people alike can therefore benefit from intentional efforts to facilitate and support genuine personal commitments. Some people make such commitments on their own. However, many people may never have a relationship with someone with a disability unless there is an organized effort that intentionally invites, facilitates and supports such a relationship. Citizen Advocacy is one such effort.

In this book, I share stories of Citizen Advocacy relationships between people with and without disabilities initiated by Citizen Advocacy programs, and I describe some of the lessons of those relationships. The stories in this book are based on personal interviews with citizen advocates and people who have advocates from the United States, Canada and Australia. In translating the spoken to the written word, I have tried to preserve the original spirit with which the words were spoken. Each advocate reviewed and sometimes edited his or her story to suggest improvements and changes.

The telling of a story by a person who lived it has an authentic ring of truth that cannot be denied. I invite you to read these stories as one on a journey, a journey of discovery and a testimony to the strength of the human spirit. I am deeply indebted to each person who shared such meaningful parts of his or her life. Following each interview, I discuss some of the lessons that struck me as I reflected on their stories.

A primary audience I have in mind is established citizen advocates who are interested in reflecting on the lessons of other citizen advocates as a way of strengthening their personal advocacy commitment. An equally important audience for this book is the people who do the work of Citizen Advocacy — the program coordinators, the board or committee members, and the support staff of local Citizen Advocacy programs. I hope that these practitioners of Citizen Advocacy will find this book helpful as they encourage citizen advocates to sustain their relationship commitments over time. The lessons of the Citizen Advocacy relationships shared in this book are also instructive for any person or group that facilitates such relationships, whether through Citizen Advocacy or through some other relationship-making enterprise. Citizen Advocacy programs have often been started by someone who became disillusioned with more formal ways of responding to vulnerable people in their communities. If this book speaks to the experience of people struggling to find a more authentic way to make a difference in the world, perhaps they are called to start a Citizen Advocacy program. This is the reason for a "why-do" book on Citizen Advocacy, a collection of lessons and insights that my colleagues and I have gleaned during my sixteen years as a Citizen Advocacy coordinator.

This book is not intended to be a recruitment tool for new advocates. While certain sections or stories may be helpful in promoting discussion with potential advocates, one cannot learn the value of a human relationship by reading a book. For that, one must be in a genuine relationship with a real human being. People need to be drawn to become citizen advocates through a genuine relationship with a real person who needs an advocate, not by a book. While an astute Citizen Advocacy Coordinator may want to share certain sections of this book with a potential advocate, much of this material will only become relevant after a Citizen Advocacy relationship is firmly established. The breadth of the issues described in this book might scare off some potential advocates, including people who over time would make excellent advocates — but at their own time, and at their own pace. Once a citizen advocate is engaged and a relationship is established, however, the insights in this book may help sustain their advocacy commitment.

Family members of a person with a disability may also find this book relevant. While Citizen Advocacy promotes voluntary, freely-chosen relationships, the personal commitments of family members to individual people with disabilities — though not necessarily freely-chosen — are among the most important relationships any person can have.

Finally, this book is for anyone who is interested in knowing how voluntary personal engagements between people with and without disabilities can transform people's lives, and for some people, change the world.

THE ROLE OF HUMAN SERVICES

When I talk with people in my community about becoming involved in the life of someone with a disability, a common response is, "Isn't there some agency that takes care of those people?" Both ordinary people and professional human service workers have fallen prey to a set of assumptions that "those people" are the sole responsibility of professional human services. As a result, ordinary citizens have been disenfranchised from, and deprived of the privilege of, having meaningful roles in the lives of people with disabilities. The notion that people with disabilities are "taken care of" exclusively by professional agencies creates invisible barriers in the minds of people with and without disabilities by creating a world of "us and them."

This is not to say that professional human services are not needed. Human services can and should support people in finding and maintaining places to live, work and learn. Relevant human services can be useful in helping people with disabilities have the kind of life that most people hope to have. However, some things — like love, commitment, fidelity and friendship — cannot be bought. As you will see in the stories in this book, money and programs cannot even guarantee safety and security.

An unfortunate consequence of expecting human services to have an all-encompassing role in the lives of people with disabilities is that ordinary citizens feel they have nothing to offer to "those people" who need "special" care. Even more tragic, the dominance of human services in people's lives conveys the message to people with disabilities that they have little or nothing to offer to typical citizens.

Citizen Advocacy challenges this notion. By creating opportunities for people to become personally engaged in one another's lives, Citizen Advocacy invites people to see beyond the disability to the person: a person who has thoughts, feelings, hopes and dreams. A person who in his essence and humanity has inherent worth and dignity.

My critique of the limits of human services does not imply that Citizen Advocacy can or should replace the human service system. Indeed, a citizen advocate may be in the role of securing appropriate services for a person, and conversely, the same citizen advocate may find ways to help the person find avenues to a better life outside of organized human services. In spite of all I will say about how human services have often failed the people they serve, high quality human services are needed and important, but only to the extent that they are part of helping people to live a good life, as opposed to having an all-encompassing, segregating, exclusive role in people's lives.

HOW THIS BOOK IS ORGANIZED

The chapters in this book are organized in a way that allows the reader — as Tom Kohler suggested in his preface — to move from concept to story and from story to concept. That is, I have intermingled the stories of Citizen Advocacy relationships with chapters on the theory and concepts behind Citizen Advocacy to give the reader a sense of how Citizen Advocacy really works. In Chapter 1, I briefly describe what Citizen Advocacy is and share a number of short Citizen Advocacy stories. I selected four stories written by people associated with Citizen Advocacy to help the reader appreciate the depth and diversity of Citizen Advocacy relationships. In Chapters 2, 3, 5, 6, 7, 9, 10, 11, 14, 17, and 18, I share stories of Citizen Advocacy relationships as told by citizen advocates. After every two or three stories is a chapter in which I describe the thought and structure of Citizen Advocacy: why Citizen Advocacy is needed (Chapter 4), the background and history of Citizen Advocacy (Chapter 8), some of the common themes and lessons of the stories shared in earlier chapters (Chapter 12), and advice and suggestions on how to effectively advocate for someone with a disability (Chapter 13).

Relationships in Citizen Advocacy do not just happen by themselves. For every relationship, there is a "story behind the story," and so in Chapter 15, I share the behind-the-scenes work that went into initiating and supporting a Citizen Advocacy relationship. In Chapter 16, I outline what I call the four "pillars" of personal engagement: human dignity, sanctity of human life, love and justice. Finally, I offer some personal reflections on relationships between people with and without disabilities, and on what those relationships can teach us about the nature of love, suffering and hope. As an appendix, I offer an overview of the principles of Citizen Advocacy (Appendix A). Appendix B contains information about where one might learn more about Citizen Advocacy programs around the world.

THE LIMITS OF THIS BOOK

Trying to do one thing well means that one should not try to do everything. Space, time, and my own limitations do not permit me to address a number of important issues in the broader disability arena. I describe the context of advocacy for devalued people, specifically within Citizen Advocacy, but I do not presume to say everything that needs to be said about advocacy or disability issues.

There has been a great deal of controversy over how we refer to "people with disabilities." Dr. Wolf Wolfensberger has written about this topic in some detail, and I agree with him that the word "disability" has seriously negative, though mostly unconscious, connotations, which space here does not permit me to address.[1] The word "handicap" has its own negative connotation, as does "retardation." I am using the term "disability," because that is the word I have used most often in my actual work in Citizen Advocacy. Most typical people have at least some understanding of what the word "disability" means, and today many people with disabilities themselves prefer "disability" to "handicap." In my Citizen Advocacy

---

[1] For a detailed discussion and treatment of the language issue, see W. Wolfensberger, *Training Institute Publication Series* (TIPS), Vol. 16, No. 6, April 1997; & Vol. 17, Nos. 1, 2, & 3, June, Aug., & Oct. 1997.

practice, I use the words "disability" and "handicap" in limited contexts and only when I need to convey that a person does indeed have an impairment. Mostly, I call people by their given names. One explanatory note on pronoun usage is that when I use the pronoun "his" or "her" it is a generic reference, including both male and female. Frequent use of "his or her" makes for cumbersome prose.

The Citizen Advocacy stories in this book, and my description of Citizen Advocacy, focus on people with physical or mental impairments — people usually referred to as having a disability. To date, Citizen Advocacy has almost entirely focused on people with disabilities, but as an advocacy form, Citizen Advocacy is applicable to any socially devalued group. Citizen Advocacy programs could, for example, be organized for prisoners, or for children who are delinquent, or for elders, or for dying people.

In this book, I concentrate on stories of long-term, committed relationships, which is what we hope for most of the time in Citizen Advocacy. However, Citizen Advocacy is designed to facilitate and support a wide range of advocacy relationships, including crisis advocates, adoption, guardianship, short-term relationships, and other kinds of relationships, depending on the life situation and needs of the person who needs an advocate. I chose to focus on long-term relationships in order to emphasize the importance of sustaining commitment over time, and to mine the depths of wisdom and insight that lasting engagements between people with and without disabilities can give us.

Ultimately, human relationships teach us as much about ourselves as they do about other people. A relationship with someone who has a disability offers lessons in life that a person may not learn in any other way. This book seeks to share those lessons through stories of life-changing, and sometimes life-saving, relationships initiated and supported by Citizen Advocacy programs around the world. In a sense, most of the stories are quite ordinary. Yet the simple ordinariness of human relationships is precisely what makes these stories extraordinary.

CHAPTER ONE

What is Citizen Advocacy?

*Citizen Advocacy is a community enterprise that arranges and sup-
ports relationships between valued, competent individual citizens and
individuals who are socially devalued[2] in our culture, usually because
of a physical or mental impairment. Citizen Advocacy organizations
bring a devalued person to the attention of a citizen who will respond
to that person's interests and needs through a freely-given relationship.
The word* advocate *means, "one who pleads the cause of another." In
Citizen Advocacy, the person who has or needs an advocate is usually referred to as a "protégé," and sometimes, as "partner."*

    *A citizen advocate, with the support of a Citizen Advocacy organ-
ization, strives to understand and represent the interests of a person
who is at risk of social devaluation as if those interests were his own.
A citizen advocate may choose to become a friend, ally, advisor, mentor, sponsor, supporter, spokesperson, protector, adoptive parent,
guardian, and/or any number of other roles in a person's life.*

    Citizen Advocacy, while fairly easy to define, is not as easy to

---

[2] The phenomenon of social devaluation, through which a person or group is
perceived as having less value than others, is described in detail in Chapter
4.

understand. People often have a number of misconceptions about Citizen Advocacy, mistaking it for an agency volunteer program, a buddy program, a legal action bureau, or a "helping the unfortunate" initiative. There is a grain of truth to all of these misperceptions, but it is a mistake to put Citizen Advocacy in a box without a more nuanced understanding of what it is. Citizen Advocacy is not one thing, but many things. A citizen advocate may help a child get into and stay in school, protect someone who lives in a nursing home, find someone a home or a job, befriend someone who has no friends, or go to court on someone's behalf. The possibilities are limitless, because each advocate's role in someone's life grows from the interests and needs of each specific person with a disability.

For centuries, the most powerful medium of transmitting cultural wisdom has been storytelling. The best way to describe Citizen Advocacy is to describe the relationships themselves, i.e., by telling their stories. It is the stories that make Citizen Advocacy alive. The full-length stories in this book are accounts of Citizen Advocacy relationships as told by advocates. They describe the ups and downs of their relationships in detail. To underscore the uniqueness and diversity of Citizen Advocacy, I first share three short stories written by people associated with the Chatham-Savannah Citizen Advocacy program in Savannah, Georgia. For more understanding of how Citizen Advocacy relationships are made, I then share a story about a relationship initiated by One to One: Citizen Advocacy in Beaver, Pennsylvania.

Sheldon and Gary[3]

by Billy Hughes

Sheldon Tenenbaum has worked for Chatham Steel for almost three decades. It's a big company, one with a well-established name in Savannah, and it would be easy to feel intimidated upon entering the lobby. After all, the receptionist is seated behind a glass partition, wired up to a switchboard. It's obvious that a visitor isn't going anywhere unless invited.

But if you take a minute to look around, the edges of this apparently formidable arrangement begin to soften. A second perusal of the lobby reveals a hefty dragon escaping from the window planter onto a carpet. It's a cheerful sight, multicolored and cast in iron, one of several metal sculptures crafted by a talented hand and subtly arranged around the room. There is more than meets the eye here, and not too far beneath the business surface. It would be difficult for Jack to become a dull boy in this place.

Life for Sheldon Tenenbaum has certainly not been dull for the past 18 years. A man named Gary Foss helped see to that. When Gary and Sheldon first met in August 1980, Gary wore out a pair of shoes a week as he pulled his legs behind him while using crutches. Gary now uses a wheelchair to get around.

And get around he does. It might not be the same stroll he used to indulge in back when Sheldon first met him, back when the small income he received went straight to an appliance store to pay for the refrigerator he bought for someone who had given him kindness. Sheldon has seen to it that Gary no longer owes his monthly check to the jeweler or the clothing store or to anyone else with an ea-zy payment plan. Managing money was one immediate need that Sheldon thought he could provide, and their first "financial conference" was held at Johnny Harris Restaurant, an air conditioned refuge from the mid-summer heat which was taking a toll on

---

[3] "Sheldon and Gary" was written by Billy Hughes, editor and publisher of *The Yokel — Local and Vocal*. Reprinted with permission from *Looking Back On The Last Twenty Years,* Chatham-Savannah Citizen Advocacy, 2000.

Gary, who had dressed in his best suit for the occasion.

But money was only the first of many issues that Sheldon and Gary grappled with together. It wasn't easy for an independent, strong willed, street-smart man like Gary to accept advice and sometimes personal help from a man he really did not know.

Temper came to play. There were arguments. Harsh words were wielded. But as the two of them came to know each other, the times got easier. Persistence proved stronger than impulse. Patience overruled anger. Both men grew and gradually learned to accept the other man's ways.

Today Gary doesn't need to worry about being bounced around from night shelter to personal care home to hospitals. He doesn't need to worry about trying to survive nursing home life again — that almost killed him the first time around. Gary receives the home-based services he needs . . . and he knows whom to call for help. Social agencies that once shunned Gary and warned Sheldon to avoid "wasting his time" now understand more about Gary.

Over time, committed allies have been found, people like Susan Earl, a woman Sheldon insists has been as much help to Gary as anyone.

Sheldon, for his part, welcomes what he has learned from knowing a man whose life he may never have chanced to consider, a life lived away from his own. The phone calls at odd hours from surprising locations for difficult reasons gave Sheldon an opportunity — to listen, to learn, and to understand a life lived under such different circumstances than his own.

As we sat together in the well-appointed office looking out over the concrete yard of the steel company, Sheldon took time to reflect on his part of this Citizen Advocacy relationship. He was matter-of-fact about the workings of their relationship, anxious to deflect any praise for what has happened. One aspect of their mutual journey made him light up: all the people who have become involved in Gary's getting along in the world. Chatham Steel employees, Sheldon's family, especially daughter Jessica (who Gary would honor yearly with a birthday gift during her growing up), and Susan Earl who has been such a big part of molding public supportive services in a way that allows for stability in Mr. Foss's home life.

Like any businessman, Sheldon cares about the bottom line. This is one ledger that shows profit all the way around.

Janie and Rachel[4]

by Rich Wittish

Janie Johnson Walker got the call to step forward as a citizen advocate one night in 1980.

Tom Kohler, the coordinator of Chatham-Savannah Citizen Advocacy, was on the phone, telling her someone was needed to befriend an 18-month-old who had been hospitalized with the diagnosis of acute brain damage from physical abuse. Tom was concerned about the toddler, whose name is Rachel, because he felt there might not be anyone from her family to watch out for her when she was in the hospital.

Earlier in the year, Kohler had visited Janie at her home to tell her about Citizen Advocacy and she seemed interested. Now he was asking her to stand up and do something that might not be possible.

Because Janie was not related to Rachel, there was a question as to whether Janie would be allowed to see her at the hospital, much less hold her and comfort her.

Janie is not certain what Tom's exact words were when he talked with her that night. "Tom probably said, 'So what if you go down there and they throw you out? This child may die if you don't go.'" said Janie during an interview from her home in Atlanta.

So she went, not knowing what to expect and not sure of what she was doing.

---

[4] "Janie and Rachel" is written by Rich Wittish, a reporter and editor for the *Savannah Morning News* for 22 years, is a locally based freelance writer and co-author of *The Insider's Guide to Savannah*. Reprinted with permission from *Looking Back On The Last Twenty Years,* Chatham-Savannah Citizen Advocacy, 2000.

"I don't know what made me decide to go, but I'm glad I did," said Janie, who was 28 at the time and managing the marketing department of the Southern Bell telephone company in Savannah.

Janie was not thrown out of the hospital that night, and she returned many times to visit Rachel, rocking the little girl in her arms and making sure that she was receiving the care she needed.

"She had such beautiful eyes . . . she was 18 months old and so huggable," said Janie of Rachel. "She was so tiny — just a baby."

"When a baby cries, everybody wants to help," she said of her relationship with the little girl. "At least I did."

Janie had won a little victory for Rachel, just by standing by her, holding her, treating her like the baby she was, but there was a bigger battle looming. She feared that when Rachel was discharged from the hospital, she would be institutionalized because her mother could not care for her and there was no one else.

Janie believed that if Rachel were placed in an institution, she would not get the attention required to insure her survival. She decided she needed to keep after the social services agency handling Rachel's situation until the agency located a home for this little girl.

During the next couple of months, Janie called the agency two or three times a week, insisting that a foster home for Rachel be found. About four months after Rachel was hospitalized, she was placed in the home of a woman named Becky Scoggins.

"Becky Scoggins is an angel," said Janie. "She took this wonderful 22-month-old baby into her home and Rachel became an integral part of her family."

When Rachel was four, Becky and her husband built a little wagon for her so she could join the other children in their play by being with them as they played around the neighborhood.

"Up until she was 12 or 13, hospitals consumed quite a bit of Rachel's time," said Janie. She feels that living through the medical problems would have been even more challenging at an institution if someone as vigilant as Becky hadn't been watching out for her. "For 18 years, Becky has gotten up twice a night to make sure Rachel was comfortable," Janie said.

Janie moved away from Savannah in 1983. It's been years since

ONE PERSON AT A TIME

362.4 Hil

	13	Mortgage insurance premiur
	14	Investment interest. Attach For
	15	Add lines 10 through 14 .
Gifts to Charity	16	Gifts by cash or check. If yo see instructions. . .
If you made a gift and got a benefit for it, see instructions.	17	Other than by cash or chec instructions. You **must** attac
	18	Carryover from prior year.
	19	Add lines 16 through 18 .
Casualty and Theft Losses	20	Casualty or theft loss(es). At
Job Expenses and Certain Miscellaneous Deductions	21	Unreimbursed employee e job education, etc. Attach (See instructions.) ▶
	22	Tax preparation fees .
	23	Other expenses—investme and amount ▶
	24	Add lines 21 through 23 .
	25	Enter amount from Form 10·
	26	Multiply line 25 by 2% (.02)
	27	Subtract line 26 from line 2·
Other Miscellaneous Deductions	28	Other—from list in instructic
Total Itemized Deductions	29	Add the amounts in the far on Form 1040, line 40 .
	30	If you elect to itemize ded deduction, check here

For Paperwork Reduction Act Notice, see Form 1·

she has seen Rachel or Becky. But she has talked with Becky long-distance on a few occasions.

Becky recently required help in having Rachel's last name changed to Scoggins, so Janie pitched in by contacting an attorney in Savannah and getting him involved in the legal maneuvering. By acting as a go-between for the family, occasionally Janie continues to get to serve as Rachel's advocate.

"It's like being an uncle who knows how to get things done," she says. "That's what I can do for Rachel now."

Al and Don[5]

by Gene Downs

Disney World trips. Movies. An occasional flash of temper. Girls calling the house. A lot of love.

Think this is an ordinary father-son-relationship? Meet Al and Don Chassereau and think again.

Al is 56, a former teacher and retired administrator for the Savannah Chatham County Board of Education. Don, who will soon be 30, is his son.

Their story starts over lunch some 16 years ago.

"I was a single person, and I had decided earlier that I was going to adopt a child," Al said. "A friend of mine at the Board of Education was going to lunch with Ann Woldt, Tom Kohler's assistant at Citizen Advocacy. Well, I went with them and mentioned that I was interested in adopting, and Ann introduced me to Tom.

"Tom is sort of like a spider. He has a web and he pulls you in — in a good way. He lures you with one of his famous lunches. So, Tom and I went out and had lunch together."

---

[5] "Al and Don" is written by Gene Downs, the arts and entertainment reporter for the *Savannah Morning News*. Reprinted with permission from *Looking Back On The Last Twenty Years*, Chatham-Savannah Citizen Advocacy, 2000.

Over sandwiches, Tom told Al about Don, a 13-year-old boy who'd been living at Georgia Regional Hospital for more than two years.

Would Al be interested in meeting Don? Of course.

At a pizza party soon afterwards, Al met Don for the first time, and things got off to a stinging start.

"He had gone to the beach the day before and was sunburned," Al remembers. "So I touched him on the shoulder, and his first reaction was one of pain.

"I thought, 'Oh, Lord, I've hurt this kid already. What an impression.'"

Procrastinating about the miles of red tape required to adopt, Al didn't follow up on the meeting.

But Tom did. And the upshot was that Al and Don began spending time together.

Their first time out, they saw "E.T." Don liked it so much, he twisted the movie's most famous line to his advantage; holding Al's hand, he'd say, "Go home" — and he wasn't talking about Georgia Regional [a state hospital].

Don met Al's family. Al's father's verdict was: "That young'un just needs love."

Al was ready to provide that, but knew that he faced plenty of bureaucratic finagling. Don's mother had released custody of Don, but his father had not. Also, the social workers had come to consider Don "unadoptable."

Still with unflagging encouragement from Citizen Advocacy, Al persevered. He met Don's caseworker at the Department of Family and Children's Services, introduced himself to Don's teachers, and generally made himself known.

On September 24, 1982, Al's patience paid off. Don went home.

"I picked him up after work, and he comes out with two grocery bags and two blue Cookie Monsters (stuffed animals), and we took him home," Al recalled, his eyes filling up at the memory.

"I was scared to death. I thought, 'What are you going to do with this young'un?' But I was just so happy. It was like bringing a baby home from the hospital."

Don lived with Al as a foster child until December 1983, when the adoption was finalized.

Al's employees threw Don a shower, members of their church embraced his new son, and friends asked how to help.

"Oh, yeah, and by the way, all hell was breaking loose at home."

"I was a biology teacher for nine years at Groves High. I knew everything about parenting — I thought," Al said.

"It was almost as if he was going to be angry enough to dissolve the relationship or prove that it would last through anything. He was testing me. Finally we calmed down."

As between any parent and child, times have not been glassy smooth, but they've been invariably rewarding.

"I realized long ago that I couldn't save the world. But I could be a father to a son," he said. "Here's my son."

And what does Don think of this?

"When I was little, I didn't have a good childhood. Till I met my daddy," he said, "Since I met him, everything's fine."

The Making of a Citizen Advocacy Relationship

The three Citizen Advocacy stories on the preceding pages should help establish that Citizen Advocacy is more than taking someone out for an ice cream cone. Citizen Advocacy is a serious relationship-making enterprise for serious people dealing with serious issues in people's lives. Citizen Advocacy is not just a friendly visiting program, nor is it any one kind of relationship. Citizen Advocacy relationships are sometimes "light" in the sense of low demand, occasional friendships. They can also be demanding, challenging, life-changing, even life-saving, relationships — and everything in between. At a 30-Year Celebration of Citizen Advocacy in Omaha, Nebraska in October, 2000, Dr. Wolf Wolfensberger, the conceptual founder of Citizen Advocacy, dubbed Citizen Advocacy the "tears and laughter" movement. Citizen Advocacy confronts the worst and brings out the best in human beings, so tears and laughter are commonplace in Citizen Advocacy relationships.

While hearing the stories of relationships helps people understand what Citizen Advocacy is, it may also help to have some understand-

ing of how Citizen Advocacy relationships come about, and how the process works. Without getting bogged down in the details of the inner workings of a Citizen Advocacy office, the following story offers some insight into how Citizen Advocacy relationships are made. This story is written by Stephen Catanzarite, a freelance writer and an associate of One to One: Citizen Advocacy in Beaver, Pennsylvania, the program of which I was a principal founder and coordinator for 16 years.

Linda and Taylor

Linda Nulph had no intention of becoming a citizen advocate. The mother of two young energetic boys, and the wife of a United Methodist minister, her life was already filled with activity and responsibility. So when One to One: Citizen Advocacy of Beaver, Pennsylvania contacted her about the possibility of becoming an advocate, Linda thought she would listen politely — and then politely decline.

"A friend gave the people at One to One my name, and Denise Shaw (the Associate Coordinator at One to One) called and asked if she could send me a video about their program. I didn't want to be rude, so I said 'yes,' but I admit I wasn't really interested," she says.

Still, Linda kept her word and watched the video, which describes the purpose of Citizen Advocacy and details three Citizen Advocacy relationships. While she was moved by what she saw, she remained reticent. "I told my husband that I was going to say no. I just didn't think I had the time to commit to something like this."

Yet when Shaw called to follow up on the video, Linda found herself agreeing to a personal meeting to discuss a little girl who needed an advocate. "I just couldn't say 'no,' " Linda recalls, laughing. "But as I was walking out the door to go to the meeting, I told my husband that, this time, I was definitely going to tell Denise that I couldn't be an advocate."

Again, however, Linda's plan to politely say "no" was foiled when, at her meeting with Shaw, she learned about a bright, spunky little girl with a radiant smile named Taylor. Taylor Cordes is the kind of person that lights up a room when she enters, and she clearly enjoys being the center of attention. Now age eight, Taylor has had cerebral palsy since birth. Though she is brimming with life and vitality, Taylor can neither walk nor talk. Despite her obvious intelligence and love for people, she has experienced the social isolation all too common for people with disabilities.

A chasm exists in our culture. There is a gulf between people with mental and physical disabilities and the rest of society. While this breach is often exacerbated by outright prejudice and discrimination, it is generally a passive sort of failing, a sad reality that goes unrecognized by people caught up in the drama of their own lives. It is a de-facto form of segregation: people who do not have disabilities rarely interact in a meaningful way with people that do. They simply don't travel in the same circles, don't live in the same places, and don't share the same experiences. The fact that societal devaluation of people with disabilities often occurs subconsciously doesn't make the situation any less tragic — or dangerous. When you compound this dilemma with our culture's deepening inability to tolerate any form of suffering, and add modern "scientific" and "philosophical" attempts to redefine the very essence of human dignity (and thus which lives are "worthy" of protection under law), the stakes are raised considerably higher.

"We find that when you take the time to explain the life experiences that are common in the lives of people with disabilities, most people are shocked and outraged," says A.J. Hildebrand, founder and coordinator of One to One: Citizen Advocacy. "The threats to people with disabilities go beyond issues of accessibility and inclusion — which we are all used to hearing about — and in some situations involve matters of life and death." Hildebrand goes on to explain that Citizen Advocacy provides a unique and potentially life-changing (and life-saving) opportunity for people to channel their outrage — and their humanity.

"By introducing two people who would otherwise not have met, and supporting those two people in a one-to-one, lasting relationship, we are essentially protecting human dignity and the rights of all people on a very fundamental level — on a personal level."

Citizen Advocacy is a sociological, not a religious, concept, and One to One and its sister programs around the world are decidedly non-sectarian. Yet at its core, the mission of Citizen Advocacy depends on the recognition that a person's dignity and rights come not from the government or any temporal ruler, but are, in fact, transcendent.

"The mission of One to One is to promote the protection of, and advocacy for, people with disabilities, not through legislation or in the court of public opinion, but through one personal relationship at a time," Hildebrand says.

In effect, Citizen Advocacy restores something to society that has been lost: true community.

The Complexity of Matching an Advocate

Talk with enough people involved, and it becomes clear that fear is probably the biggest obstacle to making and sustaining Citizen Advocacy relationships. In Linda Nulph's case, for example, fear of what would be expected of her as an advocate was a serious deterrent to saying "yes."

"I was afraid of what the expectations might be," Linda says. "I didn't want to let anybody down. I also wasn't sure how I would deal with a person's disabilities — afraid that I might say or do the wrong thing."

Of course fear is a common human emotion, and Taylor's mom, Lori, had her own concerns.

"When [the staff of One to One] told me about Linda, I was excited, but also a little nervous," Lori recalls. "The fact that Linda is a pastor's wife kind of scared me. I was afraid that, me being a single mom of two kids, she might judge me."

Lori also had a lot of apprehension about Taylor's future. She knows the time will come when Taylor will be expected to move from the school she currently attends, which caters to the needs of children with physical disabilities, to a public school.

"I have a lot of fears about Taylor moving to a public school. How will the other kids treat her? Will the teachers be sensitive to her needs? There are just a lot of questions," Lori says. At the same time, she recognizes the importance of this transition in her daughter's future.

"Taylor is very intelligent," the proud mother says. "She's an expert with the computer, and she really loves school. She loves to learn. In fact she gets mad on days when there is no school! I know she needs to be challenged and that means she needs to eventually go to a regular school. I just want to make sure the timing is right."

More than anything, however, Lori wanted an advocate who could connect with Taylor, someone with empathy who could help broaden Taylor's social circle and deepen her life experiences. Her cerebral palsy makes it difficult for Taylor to communicate, and Taylor hasn't had the opportunity to meet new people and make friends the way most other children do.

"Like a lot of parents, I've got a full-time job and another child to raise. Taylor needs a lot of attention and care, which is my responsibility," Lori says. "But she also needs to be able to see and do things that I can't always provide."

After a family member brought Lori and Taylor to a One to One social event, Lori asked Hildebrand and Shaw to find an advocate for Taylor. Before the search for an advocate could begin, however, the role an advocate would be asked to have in Taylor's life had to be clearly defined. Hildebrand and Shaw spent hours getting to know Taylor, her talent and abilities, as well as her needs and the challenges she faces. They also spent time getting to know Lori.

"When it comes to dealing with the human service system, it helps to have an ally, someone you can depend on to help you figure things out and, when necessary, speak up. A.J. and I saw right away that Taylor — and Lori — needed someone like that. Another set of eyes and ears, and another voice."

Hildebrand and Shaw decided the advocate needed to be a mother, comparable in age to Lori, who would not be afraid to stand up for what's right. After many months of searching, and one failed attempt at making a match, their search led them to Linda.

"Linda is somebody I admire," Shaw says flatly. "She has an enormous amount of energy, she's a very happy and upbeat person, and yet she understands that there is a lot wrong with the world and she wants to do something about it."

Hildebrand agrees. "We had a sense that Linda, if she agreed to being an advocate, would really commit and give it her all. The fact that she wanted to take her time and reflect on what we were asking her to do just made us respect her all the more."

After nearly two decades making and supporting matches, Hildebrand and Shaw know that the decision to become an advocate cannot be taken lightly. While they are careful not to scare a potential advocate away, they are upfront about what they are asking that person to do.

"Citizen Advocacy relationships are, in many ways, bittersweet," Hildebrand states. "We match people with a wide array of disabilities. Sometimes, we find people who are in life-threatening situations. Given the degree of devaluation such people generally experience in our society, the roles we ask advocates to assume can be challenging. We ask advocates to be life-affirming in situations that may be anything but."

Besides fear, misconceptions about what type of person it takes to be a citizen advocate can also be a stumbling block to matching. Many people think it takes an extraordinary, extra-human capacity for patience, goodness, and holiness. Just as most people never think they could end up being disabled, it seems many people think they don't have "what it takes" to be a good citizen advocate.

Some of this may be due to Citizen Advocacy's relative obscurity among other volunteer groups — an obscurity that is by design. Citizen Advocacy programs generally don't make broad appeals for volunteers or financial support via the media. This is because such appeals, though unintentionally, often lead to further stigmatization and devaluation of people with disabilities by portraying them as "pitiful" or as objects of charity. Similarly, because the work of Citizen Advocacy is to be accomplished on a personal level — one relationship at a time — generalized campaigns to "sign people up" to become advocates are not effective.

"We have to get to know people before we can match them," Hildebrand insists. "We rely on personal contacts in the communities we serve to find advocates, not on advertising campaigns or public appeals. It makes for a very slow — sometimes frustratingly slow — recruiting process, but it is the only way this work can be done right."

Yet both Hildebrand and Shaw make it clear that it doesn't take a perfect person to be a good citizen advocate.

"We're not looking for saints," Hildebrand says, "but for people who are willing to see past a disability and see a person. Beyond that, we know that nobody is perfect, and we're here to support advocates in any way we can."

Shaw echoes these sentiments: "We meet some of the best people [in our community] through Citizen Advocacy, and they are people with the same hopes, fears, hang-ups, and problems that we all deal with."

In other words, to be a citizen advocate, you have to be human. In his remarks on the 30th Anniversary of Citizen Advocacy, Dr. Wolf Wolfensberger, who in 1970 developed and helped launch the first Citizen Advocacy program in Nebraska, says "an advocate's initial motivation seems to be relatively unimportant as long as it is not dishonorable. Many advocates have started out with all sorts of strange notions and misconceptions, but have nevertheless become good advocates and learned a lot."

Taylor Cordes and Linda Nulph

Though she gave it her best shot, Linda Nulph was simply unable to say "no" to becoming a citizen advocate. And so, after much prayerful consideration, she agreed to meet Taylor Cordes and Taylor's mom, Lori.

"I knew that if I met [Taylor] there was going to be no way that I could say no, so by the time we actually met, I had my mind made up to say 'yes.'" Linda remembers. "Of course I had no idea what Taylor or Lori would think of me, and I was very nervous about that."

Lori was also nervous.

"Even with all the [human service] people we have coming to our house, it's still difficult to open your life up to someone new. I

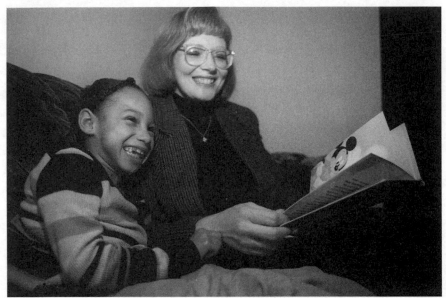

Linda and Taylor

wasn't sure what to expect," she recalls. In fact, the only person that didn't seem nervous during that first meeting was Taylor.

Described by her mom as "a people person," Taylor enjoys making new friends, and by all accounts took an instant liking to Linda.

"I believe Taylor has a certain 'gut instinct' when it comes to people, and she was just immediately comfortable with Linda," Lori says. "That gave me the reassurance I needed, and I then was able to relax," she laughs. For her part, Linda says she couldn't help but love Taylor the moment they met.

"She just has this warm smile and these big eyes and a great personality," Linda says with a warm smile of her own. "I mean, what's not to like?"

It also helped that the rapport between Linda and Lori was immediately cordial. As Lori puts it, "we just clicked."

In a relatively short time, the bond between Taylor and Linda – and between Linda and Lori – grew solid. While it is obviously important that Linda and Lori have a good and cooperative relationship, Hildebrand says Linda will always need to balance being a friend with her primary commitment to being an advocate for Taylor.

"It can be difficult for someone who is an advocate for a child, because sometimes that means going beyond what the parent feels comfortable with in terms of asking questions or making certain types of decisions" he says. "In some cases, the advocate has a better vantage point from which to see what is truly in the child's best interest, and this can potentially create a conflict between the parent and the advocate."

Linda says that, for the most part, she and Lori agree on most of the issues regarding Taylor's care, treatment, and education, and when they disagree, they are comfortable enough with each other to have an open discussion.

"One issue that we disagree over is where Taylor should attend school," Linda says. "I believe Taylor should be in a regular school learning the same things as other kids her age. But for some reasons I totally understand, Lori feels Taylor is better off in a special needs school. It's not my place to force the issue, but I think that by discussing this with Lori, it at least plants a seed for the future."

Even asking simple questions can underscore the different roles a parent and an advocate have in the life of a child with disabilities. In 2002, Linda accompanied Taylor and Lori to Children's Hospital in Pittsburgh, where Taylor underwent a complete evaluation. At the end of a long day of tests and examination, a doctor discussed treatment options for Taylor, including different types of therapies and adjustments to her medication. Linda remained in the background, quietly lending her support to Taylor and her mom. But when the doctor asked if there were any questions, Linda asked point-blank if Taylor would ever be able to walk. The doctor, in a very matter-of-fact manner, said no, and Lori burst into tears.

"I had never discussed the issue with Lori," Linda says, "and I think she preferred not knowing the answer to that particular question." Though she feels she could have handled the situation in a more delicate manner, Linda still believes that asking the question was the right thing to do because, by getting the subject out in the open, Linda and Lori were able to talk about realistic expectations for Taylor's future.

"I told Lori that there's a big difference between walking and caring for yourself — being able to stand and transfer from a chair to a bed, for example. And besides, the doctor only based his answer on statistics and his own experiences. Taylor is an individual, not a statistic."

More importantly, Linda says the episode at the hospital gave her the opportunity to see a deeper expression of Taylor's personality.

"When Lori was crying, I looked over at Taylor and saw her reaching, almost straining, to touch her mother and comfort her. It was absolutely the most beautiful thing I have ever seen." Linda adds that she feels privileged to know both Taylor and her mother, repeating a sentiment often heard from citizen advocates: "I think I get more out of the relationship than I give."

For their part, Hildebrand and Shaw both say they are grateful for the privilege of bringing Linda, Taylor, and Lori together.

"This job can be tough, filled with a lot of sadness and heartache," Shaw says. "But when you recognize the power and potential for good that a match like this one can have, it makes it all worthwhile."

CHAPTER TWO

Friends for Life:
The Story of Linda and Charlene

This chapter and the one that follows represent stories of how fidelity and human connection can grow and mature over time. Giving oneself to another human being in friendship is a precious gift. The power of two people opening themselves to one another in trust, without any pretense or threat to the continuity of friendship, cannot be overstated. The bond of a deep friendship is a safe haven against the trials and inequities of life. Following is the story of Linda and Charlene's friendship as told by the advocate, Linda Wittish.

I am the editor of *Savannah Magazine,* a regional lifestyles magazine. I am a journalist by training and graduated from Auburn University. I came to Savannah in 1974 when my husband, who is also a journalist, got a job at the *Savannah Morning News.* At the time we thought we'd come to Savannah for two or three years, get established in our careers, and then move on to a bigger paper. We fell in love with Savannah and never left. I worked at the newspaper until our daughter was born, and stayed home with her for a few years. Since then I've worked in various public relations/marketing positions — at a local college, a television station, and in health care for about 16 years. I also free-lanced for a while until the position at the magazine opened up. My husband and I have a daughter, Erica, who is now 26 and married. I also have a granddaughter, born in July 2002.

I first heard about Citizen Advocacy in 1979, over 23 years ago. A friend of mine was involved in Citizen Advocacy and was helping a family who had a child with disabilities by staying with the child from time to time. As she told me about Citizen Advocacy, I said it sounded like an interesting concept. About two weeks later, Tom Kohler called me, and we had lunch. I didn't know much about Citizen Advocacy, but it sounded intriguing. When we met, Tom said he didn't have anyone in mind to match me with at the time, but he felt sure someone would come along. Not too long after Tom called me and said he had met a woman who basically was looking for a friend outside of her circles at work and church. She wanted someone different in her life. At the time Erica was three years old; I was working part-time and involved in a lot of things, particularly at my church. I was concerned with how I would find the time. I have to say it was a scary proposition — I had never been involved in anything like this before. Tom said, "Well, let's get together, and if you and Charlene hit it off, fine, and if you don't, that's fine too."

Charlene and I are close in age; she is four years younger than me. If it weren't for Citizen Advocacy, we probably never would have met because we go to different churches and have a different circle of friends in Savannah. Charlene is visually impaired. She was born prematurely, and at that time they exposed premature babies to pure oxygen, which damaged her eyes. She had very limited vision until she was about 9 or 10 years old. She fell one day, and when she got up she couldn't see at all anymore. She has been to all kinds of doctors. When I first met Charlene, she could still distinguish light from dark, but gradually that went away too.

When we met, Charlene was single, working as a medical transcriptionist, and living in her own apartment. She has since gotten married, moved away once, bought a house, left her job, and is now taking computer classes. She lost her job as a transcriptionist when the hospital switched from typewriters to computers, but she is taking classes and thinking about getting back into the workforce.

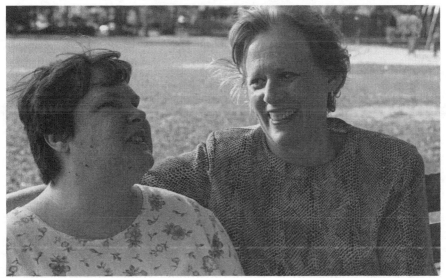

Linda and Charlene   Photograph by Ann Curry

Charlene has had a lot of difficulties in her life, and like all of us, has had her ups and downs. She attended schools for the blind, and her mother died when she was young. She is petite, very bright, and very feisty. Charlene is now happily married; her husband is also visually impaired. A few years ago they moved to Macon for a year, but they didn't like it there and moved back to an apartment here in Savannah.

One of the highlights in our relationship was when Charlene got married and she asked me to be her matron of honor. Actually, I helped her meet her husband. Charlene used to travel around Savannah on the public transit system, but she got disoriented walking home from the bus stop one day and had a run-in with the police. So she began taking cabs, and this one cab driver kept telling Charlene about this man she ought to meet. I don't remember who called whom first, but they talked by phone and agreed to meet one Saturday at a restaurant. Charlene asked me to take her to meet Albert. I realized when we got there we had no clue who we were looking for. She hadn't asked Albert what he looked like. So we walked in, sat down, and waited. There was a man sitting in the first booth with his back to us, so I went over and asked him if he was Albert. He said, "Yes," and so they got together. I stayed a little while and left. Less than a year later, they got married, and it was a joyous occasion.

My relationship with Charlene has been an interesting journey. It has really been about friendship. We haven't done any of those tremendous, heroic, fighting the state legislature kinds of advocacy; it has just been a slow, steady friendship, seeing each other through the good times and the bad. We pick up the phone and call one another. I guess one of my roles in Charlene's life is that I am someone she can bounce ideas off of, like if they are thinking about a big change or something. I am someone she can talk to. She can say anything she feels she needs to say. We can sit and talk over lunch, and she will tell me things that she may not tell anyone else. Over the years, that seems to have been a help, just to have somebody to listen.

As we get older, we're thinking about what's down the road. Charlene's husband has been having some medical problems, and lately we have been talking about how they can maintain their independence, live the way they would like, and still deal with day-to-day challenges. So we discuss options.

I always knew Charlene was, and is, a strong person. She is so resilient. Things don't always work out the way she hopes, but she always bounces back. She is amazingly supportive of other people, particularly people going through some of the same struggles she is. She is a great support to them, but she sometimes underestimates her own strengths.

I have often wondered if I had walked in her shoes and lived the life she's had, how well would I be doing? I have only had a glimpse of what her life has been like. For example, when I am with Charlene, people often talk as if she isn't there. I remember the time we went to the bank to deposit Charlene's check, and the teller looked at me and asked, "What does she want to do with it?" I said, "I don't know; why don't you ask her?" People mean well, and they are not trying to be hurtful, but they are either intimidated by or uncomfortable with someone who has a disability, and they don't know how to react. They either over-react or don't react at all. That happens frequently in restaurants and in other public places.

What stands out in our relationship is the fact that we have stuck together so long. We have shared joys and sorrows. Like when my daughter got married, or when there was illness in my family, Charlene was the one who was supporting and comforting me. When Charlene lived away for a year, it was a real adjustment for both of us. We missed one another. Except for my husband and my family, I have had a consistent relationship with Charlene longer than anyone. People come into your life, and there may be a very concentrated relationship for a while, but then you drift apart. Twenty-three years is a long time, and I cannot think of anyone else with whom I have made a conscious effort to consistently keep up a friendship for that long.

One of the great benefits of my friendship with Charlene is that my daughter Erica has grown up with her. As a child, Erica never had any reservations about being around someone with a disability. As she has grown up, she has come in contact with other people with disabilities, and she is not at all intimidated or shy. Erica always went to the grocery store with us, and she would anticipate Charlene's needs almost before she spoke. Erica is a more well-rounded person because of having known Charlene. In high school, she wrote a paper about inclusive education, and she graduated from college with a degree in learning disorders. Now she teaches children who have problems learning in traditional ways. I think her interest in helping people with disabilities has something to do with having been around Charlene.

I have learned a great deal from Charlene. I always tell Tom that I get much more out of the relationship than I give. I have become more tolerant of people, and I have a clearer understanding of discrimination. Citizen Advocacy has helped me recognize some of my own subtle prejudices. A lot of pre-conceived notions I had have been peeled away. I'm not there yet, but I feel like I am a better person for having known Charlene. I try not to make judgments about people. Maybe that is because your perspective changes as you get older, but I believe a good bit of it is because of my relationship with Charlene.

When you have a long-term relationship with someone, when you feel totally comfortable with that person, when you feel like you can be whoever you are and you can say whatever you want to say, that is a gift. It grounds you and helps you look beyond your-self and think more about other people. It helps you think about how you act, how you speak, and about what kind of impact you have on others.

Charlene's greatest gift to me is her friendship. She gives me her time. She is always willing to listen. She is a very loyal, forgiving person. Her willingness to trust is amazing. There are not many people who are willing to allow you to show all of yourself — the good, the bad, and everything in between. I can say anything to Charlene, and she would never think I was an awful person and end the relationship. To have someone who is going to stick with you no matter what — that is a real gift.

Author's Comments

Linda and Charlene's relationship illustrates a number of strong ratio-nales for Citizen Advocacy. Had there not been a Citizen Advocacy program in Savannah, it is likely that Linda and Charlene never would have met. The social circles that people with and without dis-abilities travel in tend to be separate. Many people with disabilities do not even have a social circle in which to travel. Overcoming social barriers calls for an intentional way of bringing people together in relationships. Yet most people do not become connected to one anoth-er through a relationship-making enterprise. One could argue that Citizen Advocacy is an artificial way for people to get to know one another. In other contexts, we encounter "match-makers" — people who intentionally introduce people — such as executive placement services, university mentors, and the wise yentas who in some cultures arrange marriages.

Advocates and people who have advocates often find the match-making feature of Citizen Advocacy a little awkward at first, but gen-erally find their own way in establishing genuine bonds that supersede the artificial manner in which they were introduced. Over time, the role of the Citizen Advocacy office in facilitating the relationship fades into the background, and the relationship takes on a life of its own.

Linda's relationship with Charlene points to another reason for having a Citizen Advocacy program. As Linda describes, she was — and is — a busy person. Sometimes busy people respond to a vulnerable person in their neighborhood, church, place of employment or other gathering place without being asked. In spite of their busy lives they make room for people outside their normal circles of friends and family. However, many people may not be so inclined, and need to be asked to get involved.

A number of social thinkers have concluded that positive social change only happens through relationships.[6] That is, unless a social endeavor is based on genuine relationships, that endeavor is not likely to have much effect. Linda and Charlene found a place in one another's lives that no other person can fill. Rather than rely solely on a human service system to solve problems, Charlene has a friend whom she can count on for advice and support in solving her own problems.

---

[6] See, for example, McKnight, J. (1995). *The careless society: Community and its counterfeits.* New York: Basic Books. pp.119-122. See also Schwartz, D. (1992). *Crossing the river: Creating a conceptual revolution in community and disability.* Cambridge, MA: Brookline Books. pp. 174-182.

CHAPTER THREE

"We Got Him Out": The Story of Rick and Darryl

Denise Shaw and I initiated and supported Rick and Darryl's relationship at One to One: Citizen Advocacy. The lessons and insights we learned from their story span 16 years. The ups and downs of Rick and Darryl's relationship include times of victory, failure, and everything in between. Through it all, Rick's humility and perseverance in the face of many obstacles inspired us time and again. Following is Rick and Darryl's story as told by Rick Sheffield, the advocate.

I am the seventeenth of eighteen children, the youngest boy! We grew up in a family with a lot of love. My father was a preacher, and he died when I was young; I was thirteen. My mother was the backbone of our family — she taught us quite a bit. Most all the kids in our family, I think sixteen of them, are college graduates. When you come from a big family, the idea of family is always there in the background. My wife and I have twin boys and a little girl. My father always taught us that you have to give something back — you shouldn't just be taking — you have to give things back to the community. So when the opportunity came along to do something with Darryl, it automatically clicked.

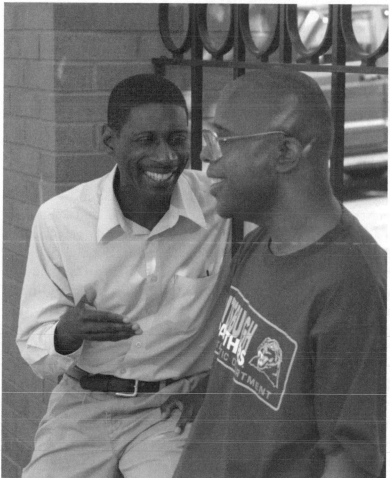

Rick and Darryl

Darryl's parents were divorced, and his mother had a tough time raising him. Darryl has a handicapped brother who was in an institution and is now in a group home. When I met Darryl, it was just he and his mother. He was fourteen when we met — raw energy. At first I had a hard time communicating with Darryl. I would say, "Darryl, how you doing today?" He'd say, "Hi." Or I'd say, "Darryl, do you want some pop?" He'd say, "pop." He never talked in sentences. Sometimes even his mother couldn't understand him.

Darryl is severely mentally handicapped as a result of brain damage during birth. They said he might be schizophrenic, because he goes around holding his ears most of the time — but he only does this because noise tends to bother him. Darryl is a little intimidating when you first see him, because he's heavy set and tall.

When we started, we did a lot of things: bowling, miniature golf, and things like that. I often brought my nephews along who were around the same age. I tried to get Darryl involved in the family with young people his age. One time we went bowling and one of my nephews was acting up so I had to say something to him. I had to yell at my nephew. Darryl thought that was pretty funny.

We did a lot of things around the house, or we'd just sit and spend time together. Most of the time I took him to family functions or to other things I was doing. I coached basketball, and sometimes he went to practice with me. I'd ask him, "What do you want to eat?" He would say, "Hot Dog Shoppe," or "McDonald's." If you asked him, "What do you want to do, Darryl?" He'd say, "golf," or "bowling." Sometimes it was like pulling teeth trying to get him to talk. But the relationship has grown. In the beginning I saw him about once a week. Later on, it got to the point where it was almost every day. A couple of times he was in a crisis — he was institutionalized twice — so I had to be in close contact with him because things became unstable in his life.

Darryl's mother was having a hard time with Darryl. She would have the TV on, for example, and Darryl didn't like it because it was too loud for him. He would go to his room saying, "noise bothering me." Or he'd leave the apartment and go to the manager's office, which was next door to his apartment. If his mother wasn't home the apartment manager would call and ask me to come down. I gave them my number in case anything happened with Darryl or his mother.

His mother did the best she could, but she didn't really know what to do with Darryl. She was having problems of her own and was on a fixed income. Darryl was in school during the day, but was home in the evening. His mother had a "sitter" through a respite care program, but she was only allotted so many hours, which she'd use up pretty fast. When she wanted to do something or wanted some time to herself, she'd call me, so I was seeing Darryl pretty often.

When Darryl was about eighteen years old, Darryl's mother was starting to become frustrated. Darryl was holding his ears a lot, and at one point, Darryl was put into a mental hospital. He kept holding his ears, and they had him on several different kinds of medications. They institutionalized him for a while. They kept saying, "we're evaluating, we're evaluating, we're evaluating." They could only keep him in the local mental health center for so long, and so a hearing came up to decide about sending Darryl to the State Hospital. I knew that wasn't the place for Darryl. He just needed someone to take a little time with him, and he'd be fine. But I really got a rude awakening.

When his mother and I went to the hearing, we learned that the decision had already been made. Without any real discussion or debate, the decision was, "We're sending Darryl to the state hospital." I thought I failed him as an advocate. They never offered me the opportunity to say anything. The lawyer who spoke on Darryl's behalf had said, "Yeah, we're going to give you a chance [to speak]." But all he did was say, "I agree."

We went up to see Darryl at the state hospital, and the conditions were deplorable. His clothes were soiled; his hair was all messed up. I took his mother up there and she looked at him. I said, "You see what the situation is?" She said, "Yes." I said, "Now, let's do whatever we can to get him back home. We'll get him into a situation that's best for him and for you." She agreed.

They said he was hearing voices. Everyone made a big deal of that. Once we decided to get him out of there and move him back home, we had to ask ourselves what the best scenario might be. His mother and I thought that maybe coming back home isn't what's best; maybe we could find a group home close by, which is what ended up happening.

I told the doctors and the caseworkers I wasn't satisfied with the conditions he was living in at the state hospital. I told them about the things I saw. If no one had said anything, he'd probably still be up there. Someone had to say something. When he came back, we were able to get him into a group home. First he was in a place several miles away, then we got him transferred to New Brighton, not too far from his mother, and not too far from me. There are less people there, and he's closer to his mother. I ride my bike past there all the time, so I usually stop in to see how he's doing. Things are calmer now, so there's not as much disruption in his life like it was during the first five or six years after we met. With young kids at home, my life has changed where I can't do as much with Darryl as I used to. I'm glad we got him into a situation that's stable.

We've had some minor problems at the sheltered workshop. He was having some trouble there and they had to cut back his hours for a while, but we worked things out and now his hours are back to normal. Sometimes people don't understand Darryl's actions, so I try to explain his behavior the best I can. I try to help them see what he is saying by his behavior. Things are pretty stable now.

I think if I hadn't met Darryl through Citizen Advocacy, Darryl would definitely be institutionalized. I think I helped bring him out of his shell. When I first met Darryl, he would just sit and rock. Once he started hanging around my nephews, playing basketball and doing things, he became more relaxed. When we go out golfing, he knows when it's his turn. Or when we go bowling, my nephews will say, "slap me five!" And he gives them five, and he knows when he does something new and he'll go slap them five again. Instead of saying, "pop," now he says, "Coke."

Darryl has brought a lot into my life. He has brought just as much to me as I have to him. Seeing the progress he made in school and talking to his teachers made me feel good. I was always there for his plays. He took part in plays, and I would watch him out there on the stage. He has grown from when I first met him. In the end, I got a lot of happiness. I'm happy about the things I've done for Darryl. When you're in the middle of things, you don't think about what you're doing at the time. Sometimes things just need to be done immediately, and you just do it, you don't worry about it.

I think I have been able to get Darryl's viewpoint across to people, as if I was speaking through Darryl. I try to put myself in Darryl's shoes to get his point of view across. I think the people at the group home and at the sheltered workshop understood that a little bit. I probably also helped Darryl's mother realize some of Darryl's needs. With other people, I don't know if I made a big difference. I try to help people avoid judging Darryl, to stop and think before jumping to conclusions.

The hardest part was when they put him in that institution. That hurt. I felt I had failed him. He was there a good three months. Darryl had become a part of me. It was almost as if they were taking my son, someone I had grown to love. I had been with him, and I knew some of the things they were saying about him weren't true. Sometimes I doubted myself — they were doctors and nurses — but then I thought, "Is this just the system not working?" I thought, "No, the system has to be wrong, this isn't fair." I understood what was going on. I felt I was the only one on his side. In the long run it worked out. We were praying about it. We got him out of there. Darryl doesn't belong in an institution. He needs to be in a place where someone cares and gives him attention. I don't think Darryl will ever be able to be on his own. I'll need to keep in touch, to stay involved and see that his life goes all right, and that no one takes advantage of him. There were times when I'd question myself. I'd ask myself, "Can I do this?" I didn't mind giving my time. Sometimes it was a juggling act with my family, but things always seemed to work out.

When you think about it, there must be more Darryls out there. You know you can't save the world, but everyone should have a fair chance, at least an opportunity, to be happy.

Author's Comments

A concept rich with meaning in Citizen Advocacy is that of identification. Andy Baxter says that identification means, "to be one with in thought or action."[7] Rick became an advocate for Darryl because he put himself in Darryl's shoes. He imagined himself as a young teenager without a father around, no extended family nearby, and no friends — a sharp contrast to Rick's childhood. Rick imagined being teased and taunted by children in the neighborhood. He thought of a single

---

[7] Baxter, A. (2002). Interpreting a Human Being. *Citizen Advocacy Forum,* 12(1 & 2), 32-50.

mom trying to hold things together in the face of an uncertain future. And he cried.

Rick felt compassion, a word that comes from the Latin com, meaning, "to be with," and passio, meaning "feeling, suffering." Identifying with Darryl and his situation moved Rick's heart. Most often, this is what brings advocates to act — a movement in one's heart. Sometimes it is a sense of justice that moves people, but for Rick, it was his heart that moved him to act.

Rick's relationship with Darryl helped save Darryl from life in an institution. If not for Rick, Darryl would most likely today be staring at cement walls and tile floors. Yet Rick's involvement with Darryl did not start out as heavy-duty advocacy. Rick and Darryl were going along fine until events transformed their relationship from simple friendship to vigorous advocacy — a common occurrence in Citizen Advocacy.

When Darryl was institutionalized, Rick did what he had to do. He knew one of the mental health caseworkers from his family connections, so he was able to give the caseworker a context for what was going on with Darryl. His first step was to help Darryl and his mother see one another. Then he convinced the social workers and the doctors that Darryl could and should return home.

Without Rick, Darryl most likely would have ended up as a long-term patient in a state hospital, lost in the bowels of the mental health system. Yet Rick is uncomfortable with being thought of as a hero. What he did was not heroic, but ordinary. Telling a caseworker that a mother loves her son is an ordinary thing to say. Buying a loaf of bread for Darryl's mom on the way home and having a friendly chat are ordinary things to do. For Rick, treating someone like family is an ordinary way to be. As Rick says, "All you really need to be an advocate is a good heart. You don't need special training, Ph.D.s, or things like that. You just treat the person as you would treat someone in your family, like a sister or a brother or a mother or a father."

Rick's advocacy on Darryl's behalf was not inspired by a social change agenda, or by deep philosophical thoughts, or even by training in advocacy. Rick simply did what his common sense and his good heart told him to do. Darryl is like a son to Rick, and fathers want their children to have the best life possible.

Rick's relationship with Darryl has weathered many storms. Advocates often go through struggles that make it hard to maintain their involvement. A crucial difference between Citizen Advocacy and other forms of advocacy is that most of the time, citizen advocates are asked to form lasting relationships. Sometimes, Citizen Advocacy relationships last for life. This dimension of Citizen Advocacy is crucially important, because human problems are not just for the moment, isolated and separated from the past or future.

As we support advocates through difficult times, we have learned that "winning" is not the most important thing, but perseverance. When Rick thought he had lost Darryl to the institution, he cried, and we cried with him. In situations like that, words fail. What do you say when someone's heart is broken? I admit that at the time I was thinking, "Citizen Advocacy is not enough. The problem is bigger than we are." We did not have a solution. All we could give Rick was our support, our presence, and our prayers. Rick is very clear that his faith is what kept him going through all the trials and tribulations in Darryl's life.

After 16 years, Rick describes Darryl as happy. The contrast between sitting huddled in a corner in a psychiatrically-drugged fog in a state hospital, and sitting at a local restaurant over a hamburger and French fries, joking and laughing with Rick, is a testimony to the triumph of faith and the power of love.

CHAPTER FOUR

Why Citizen Advocacy is Needed:
The Effects of Social Devaluation

In the early 1990s I was asked to give a presentation on Citizen Advocacy at a conference on disability issues in Washington, DC. Almost 2,000 people, mostly professional human service workers, some family members of people with disabilities, and a few people with disabilities, attended the conference. On the first day, the keynote speaker stepped up to the microphone and proclaimed, "I am here to announce that the revolution has come. Look around you. Look at all the people here. It's happened. The new revolution of inclusion and equal opportunity is here!" Everyone clapped wildly. I sat there and thought, "Well, if there was a revolution, it passed over my hometown."

Day in and day out I learn of people who have missed out on this "revolution." I meet people who are lonely, excluded, abandoned, oppressed, drugged, and sometimes, hastened to death. This is a reality that most people do not want to hear. I don't blame them. Who wants to hear about bad things happening to vulnerable people right in their own community? I don't want to hear such things, let alone say them. But after 30 years of working with people with disabilities in my community, I have to say that many, many people with disabilities remain set apart, isolated and sometimes, abandoned. I have had the opportunity to visit various human services and many Citizen Advocacy programs throughout the United States, Canada and Australia, and I find the situation in other locales pretty much the same. If a revolution has happened, it has been mostly for the human service workers, not the people being served.

It is true that there have been vast improvements in services for people with disabilities since the "snake-pit" days of massive institutions. It is also true that some people with disabilities have more physical access to the world around them through improved transportation and housing. Community programs that help people live fairly typical lives abound. Some schools are promoting inclusion for children with disabilities who in past years might not even have lived, let alone gone to school. I was part of the deinstitutionalization movement in the 1970s and 1980s that brought a substantial number of people back to their home communities to find a better life. Many positive things have happened and are happening for people with disabilities, which I applaud and support. However, my colleagues in Citizen Advocacy and I continue to meet people whose lives are untouched by the "normalization / community-building / inclusion / social participation / self-determination / no labels / Americans with Disabilities Act" revolution.

A major part of our work in Citizen Advocacy has been listening to the stories of individual people with disabilities, and sharing those stories with citizens in the community. Following are brief vignettes about just a few of the people whose lives remain untouched by the "revolution" in human services:

- George, a man who lived in a state institution during his childhood, moved into a group home, but had difficulty living with other mentally retarded people. He now lives in a boarding home with 20 elderly people. After millions of dollars have been spent on his life, he has a small corner of a bedroom that he shares with three other men. His possessions consist of a nightstand, a single bed, a few clothes, and a broken radio.

- Alex, a mentally retarded man who moved out of an institution to live in a group home, died from an infection that was complicated by hepatitis. The group home staff was unaware of his history of hepatitis, because records from the institution were shoddy and incomplete. Had it been known he had hepatitis, Alex might still be alive.

• John, a teenager who suffered a severe brain stem injury from a drunk-driving accident, was described as being in a "persistent vegetative state." When his medical insurance ran out, he was transferred to a hospice facility where his food and water were withdrawn, causing him to dehydrate and starve to death.

• Eleanor lived in a supervised apartment for years until she fell and could not walk anymore. She now lives in a large nursing home. Every time I see her, she begins to cry and says, "Can I please go back to my apartment? I don't want to live here."

• When Kim, a young woman with Down's syndrome, was five years old, she had a severe lung infection and her mother brought her to the emergency room for treatment. Standing in the hallway, her mother overheard the emergency physician say to a nurse: "Don't worry about this one, she has two normal sisters at home."

• Mallory, an eleven-year-old who has multiple disabilities, had a life-threatening infection and her mother took her to the emergency room for treatment. The emergency room doctor pulled the mother aside and asked, "How much do you want us to do, given her 'quality of life'?"

• Margaret is in her mid-fifties, has severe mental retardation and has lived in a boarding home for at least the last five years. None of her caretakers knows where she is from or if she has any family. One caretaker told us: "She doesn't understand anything." After visiting a while, we mentioned it was time to leave, and Margaret got up from her chair and showed us to the door.

• A woman with Down's syndrome had an intestinal blockage and was unable to eat. She required intravenous lines and tube feeding to sustain her until the blockage could be removed. The physician at first refused to administer tube feeding, and was prepared to starve her to death until the woman's sister insisted that a feeding tube be inserted and that the intestinal problem be corrected.

- In a one month period in the mid-1990s we talked with five different young couples who told us that they had been advised by doctors to institutionalize their child and "get on with their lives" — something we thought had happened only in the 1950s and 1960s, not the 1990s.

In our little Citizen Advocacy program in Beaver, Pennsylvania, we hear many stories like these on a regular basis. My Citizen Advocacy colleagues around the world see and hear similar stories all the time. To the people in these stories, it is beside the point whether things are any better or worse overall for people with disabilities; but I know what I see, and I know what many others are seeing.

The Nature of Social Devaluation[8]

To "devalue" someone means that consciously or unconsciously, one person perceives another as being less valuable, less worthy, less important, less a person, or even as less than human. Devaluing attitudes are usually unconscious, since most of us do not want to

---

[8] I attribute most of my understanding of social devaluation to the work of Dr. Wolf Wolfensberger, Susan Thomas and Darcy Elks. The Training Institute for Human Service Planning, Leadership, and Change Agentry at Syracuse University, directed by Dr. Wolfensberger, has developed trainers around the world who teach what social devaluation is and how it affects devalued people through a presentation called "The Most Common Life Experiences ('Wounds') of Devalued (Especially Handicapped) People." This presentation and its variations might be thought of as the collective story of the lives of devalued people, as it describes the patterns of wounding life experiences that overwhelmingly and systematically befall devalued people. The Training Institute may be contacted at 800 S. Wilbur Ave., Suite 3B1, Syracuse, NY, 13204. Phone: (315) 473-2978.

admit that we regard some human beings as less valuable than ourselves. The truth is, we all devalue somebody, at least to some degree. Consciously or not, we make negative judgments about people who have characteristics we do not value.

Social valuation is defined by the norms and values of a culture. Our society places high value on health, wealth, beauty, youthfulness, productivity, intelligence, achievement, pleasure, convenience and personal autonomy, so it follows that we are inclined to devalue anyone who is, or is perceived as, sick, poor, unbeautiful, old, "lazy," "stupid," a failure, inconvenient and/or as interfering with our enjoyment and choices in life. The people most likely to be devalued are people who are chronically ill, dying, elderly, unemployed, mentally handicapped or disordered, homeless, difficult to be with, or anyone who makes inconvenient or challenging demands.

A friend of mine whose son has a physical disability helped me appreciate the meaning of the word "devalue." During one of our many discussions about what is going on in the world, he said, "You know, that word, 'devalue,' is a heavy word." What struck me about his comment was not what he said, but how he said it. I could see in his eyes that saying the word "devalue" was painful. To think that some people would not consider his son to be as valuable as other people because of his disability must create deep personal anguish—as it would for any parent. I understand, then, why some people resist thinking about social devaluation. It is crucial, however, that allies of devalued people understand the impact that devaluing thoughts, words and actions can have. As a result of social devaluation, many people are pushed to the margins of our communities, and subjected to a pattern of harmful life experiences. If we are going to do anything about social devaluation, it is not enough to know that it exists; we must know why it exists and what its effects are.

The Impact of Social Devaluation

Social devaluation separates and divides people. Once separated, devaluing attitudes can have devastating impact. Jean

Vanier[9] speaks of the ways in which devalued people have been hurt as "wounds." A wound is a serious injury inflicted from the outside, and is deeply felt. To be wounded means a person has been violated, and perhaps repeatedly so. All of us experience some degree of emotional, psychological, or spiritual wounds in our life-time. We sometimes hear this idea of woundedness referred to as "emotional scars," "psychological trauma," or "wounded souls." Non-physical wounds can do even more damage than physical ones. A psychological or spiritual trauma, such as a broken relationship, the breach of a sacred trust, or the loss of a loved one can be so pro-found that it disrupts every aspect of a person's life.

By definition, a physical or mental impairment tends to make life more difficult by limiting a person's capacity to function. Even more limiting, however, is the negative social response that people tend to have towards people with physical or mental impairments. People with disabilities need support, adaptation and accommoda-tion in order to function in certain areas of life. Yet the social dis-tance between people with and without disabilities creates barriers to such support.

People who have even minor impairments frequently experience social and physical barriers that prevent interaction and friend-ships. I once interviewed a man who had an impairment that affected his facial appearance, and he described what it is like to deal with people's reaction to his appearance every day. At one point in our conversation, he looked into my eyes and said, "Sometimes I think I am in Hell."

The rejection that devalued people experience in life can be mild and subtle, or it can be extreme and overt. Rejection takes many forms, from being the last child picked for a sports team, to never having a date, to never having a friend, to being denied the right to go to a neighborhood school, to being sent away to an institution, to being denied adequate medical treatment. Some people, such as a person living on the street, may even be called a "reject." Everyone

---

[9] Jean Vanier is the founder of L'Arche, a network of intentional communities around the world in which people with and without disabilities live togeth-er in communal homes and share their lives.

experiences rejection in life, but devalued people are often rejected over and over again by significant people in their lives and by society, and may never find unconditional acceptance by anyone, even from their families.

We must not delude ourselves into thinking that segregation is a thing of the past. While opportunities for physical and social integration of devalued people into community life have improved, segregation still exists in all of our communities. In the United States, thousands of people with disabilities have been "deinstitutionalized" into group homes, boarding homes, and other public and private facilities that are largely segregated from the valued community. The fact that people's living quarters are closer to the general population does not by itself preclude their segregation from typical people in the community. A mile from where I live is a large nursing home where over 600 people, including many with disabilities, sit in their chairs or lay in their beds for endless hours, waiting to die. Ironically, this huge facility tends to be "less worse" than some of the smaller boarding homes and personal care homes I have seen, places in which, as one citizen advocate put it, "I would not put my dog." In my community of 180,000, I estimate that there are close to 3,000 people, most of them elderly but including many people with disabilities, living in some type of segregated setting.

Partly because of physical segregation, people with disabilities typically do not have the same opportunities to develop relationships as people who have socially valued qualities and characteristics. This is especially true when natural relationships are driven out by a preponderance of paid professional relationships. As one mentally handicapped man who had spent most of his life in human service settings described: "In my world, there are two kinds of people — clients and staff."

Devalued people often experience their social world as a kind of relationship "circus," where people come and go like actors on a stage. In many human service settings, it is not unusual to hear of staff turnover rates of 50%, 100%, or even 400% in a single year. Imagine being a person with a physical impairment who must rely on others for physical care, and having fifty pairs of hands touching you in a month's time. With so many people coming and going, and most of them only present as long as they are paid, many devalued people have never had the experience of a genuine, lasting, personal relationship.

Some people living in human service settings get moved repeatedly, agency to agency, program to program, class to class, group home to group home, institution to institution. One young woman I know had lived in over thirty different foster homes, mental health facilities, and institutions by the time she was 16. She had experienced so much rejection that, when I met her, she was almost unreachable and extremely difficult to be around. She had attempted suicide a number of times, and had set fires in several places as a way to get transferred somewhere else.

As a result of the types of experiences I have described, many socially devalued people are alone in the world, and have lost most or all of their natural, freely-given relationships. Compared to the social network that valued people typically have, the social world of devalued people is usually quite stark. There may be few, if any, unpaid people in a person's life, and even fewer whom the person can count on over time. The impact of such abandonment makes people feel unworthy, unloved and unlovable.

A major consequence of this repetitive breakdown of relationships is its impact on a person's ability to trust. Whether or not one was loved, held and cherished during one's formative years has profound consequences in a person's life. A child who has lived in an institution or other settings apart from a loving family misses the opportunity to develop the bonds of trusting relationships that influence how he understands the world and himself.

Most socially devalued people have been systematically and continuously wounded by exclusion, rejection, and segregation throughout the course of their lives. One could say that for them, social devaluation is life-defining. Not only are devalued people more likely to be wounded, but also additional wounds, even "small" ones, tend to have greater impact. These experiences, and the fact that they are likely to be repeated, cause people to exist in a state of heightened vulnerability. Valued people usually have access to resources — friends, family, and money — that help them cope with wounds in life. Someone who lives in a state of heightened vulnerability, however, typically has few resources with which to cope, and thus may have great difficulty dealing with hurtful experiences. When a devalued person is wounded one more time, we can say that another brick is added to what may already be a heavy load of systematic and relentless wounding experiences.

Wounds can heal, but only when given the opportunity. Some may never heal entirely, in which case one must learn to live with them. Bearing such wounds will often require a great deal of support from people who are genuinely committed to standing by a wounded person. Those who do not find healing, or who cannot adapt to the wounds of their past, may face great suffering and anguish for the rest of their lives.

The Problem of Patterned, Systematic Devaluation in Human Services

Appreciating the systematic, pervasive nature of social devaluation is a challenge many people are simply unable or unwilling to face. Such people are more likely to regard the difficulties that devalued people face in life as due to unfortunate circumstances rather than resulting from patterned and systematic social devaluation. However, social devaluation is not accidental, and it is more than just unfortunate circumstances. It springs from the values a culture embraces. Discerning the patterns of social devaluation forces one to address some fundamental questions about the world and the people who live in it.

Social devaluation is made worse by fear — fear of the unknown, fear of difference, fear of vulnerability and weakness. People tend to be afraid of what they do not understand. Many people have a visceral reaction to human impairment, especially if the impairment is significant. Physical and mental impairments are subtle reminders to able-bodied people that we are all imperfect, and we are all mortal. Most people acquire one or more impairments of some degree before they die, and of course every one of us will die. Human impairment is a sign of our mortality, a reminder that sooner or later, we all become frail and die. This creates fear, and we distance ourselves from people who elicit those fears.

Our society has accommodated these fears by creating segregated client worlds for people with disabilities. Since about 1960, a professional sub-culture has developed which has defined people with disabilities as needing agency-centered care. Two generations have grown up with the myth that people with disabilities need to be "taken care of" solely by professionals.

Professional competence can be valuable for certain needs. For example, if one has a problem with mobility, it is helpful to have someone who is an expert on adaptive mobility equipment bring his expertise to bear on the problem. If someone is having difficulty finding gainful employment, training to develop the person's competency and capacity for work is important. A family who has a child with complex medical needs can often benefit from supportive nursing care in the family's home.

However, when professional services usurp the prerogative, and the responsibility, for responding to needs that by definition must be met through freely-given relationships, we have a problem. The most basic human need is for love. Love cannot be bought and paid for, nor can it be forced. Love can neither be a requirement nor a duty in a job description. Love cannot be prescribed. Love can only come from one heart to another — person to person. This may sound trite, but it's true. All people need friends, not just friendly staff. We all need a home, not a place that is merely home-like. We all need something meaningful to do, not "simulated work" or "work therapy." How do most people find friends, a home, or something meaningful to do? Through people who are a part of their lives — family, neighbors, friends, and acquaintances. Obviously, we all want people in our lives who are there because they love us for who we are. We need to take the obvious seriously.

Many people in our culture have become subtly convinced that people with disabilities need to live in separate places, ride on separate vans, go to separate activities, and live in a separate world. People with disabilities — especially those who have both physical and mental impairments — become seen as so different that many ordinary experiences, such as having a friend, owning a house, having a job, or learning how to read, are not expected to happen. Without a positive vision of what life might hold for a person with a disability, service providers, families, neighbors — and sadly, even people with disabilities themselves — become accustomed to lowered expectations about what might be possible.

One of the most common experiences of devalued people is waiting — waiting for a call back from a social service agency, waiting for someone to decide on one's eligibility for services, waiting for funds to be allocated. People who live in nursing homes spend most of their time waiting to die. Young people with disabilities who live in nursing homes may wait for death their entire lives.

The combination of dynamics described above results in the disenfranchisement of people with and without disabilities. People with disabilities are seen as powerless "clients" who must have programs administered to them. Neighbors and friends are seen as not qualified and not able to do anything relevant in the life of a person who has a physical or mental impairment. The mythology of a professional sub-culture develops its own language and fancy acronyms that convince families, neighbors, and people with disabilities that their world must forever be a world of diagnoses, labels, social workers, therapists, counselors, aides, doctors, residential caretakers, and so on.

When people with disabilities live in a clientized world, routines and roles become established. The expectations of "client" and "staff" compel people to act in ways that are consistent with their prescribed role. Anyone who deviates from these expectations is at risk of being punished — either overtly or covertly. For example, someone who refuses to screw nuts and bolts together day after day at an activity program or sheltered workshop may be seen as "noncompliant." Someone who is expressing anguish over never having been loved may be interpreted as psychotic. Staff members who step out of their professional roles in response to such people are cautioned against "getting too close to the clients" and told to keep their "objectivity" or their "therapeutic distance."

Human relationships do not happen in a vacuum, and they are subject to the myriad of social forces I have described. These forces, both in the world and within the human heart, prevent, break down and destroy genuine personal relationships.

Threats to the Lives of Devalued People

The ultimate physical and social distance that can be imposed on devalued people is to literally kill them, if not directly, then indirectly by hastening their deaths. We are now in a time and age, since about 1970, in which extensive, hidden killings of thousands of people with disabilities — in reality a new genocide — is taking place. Dr. Wolfensberger has been warning us about this genocide since about 1975, but few have heeded his warning. Those who ally themselves with devalued and vulnerable people, however, will sooner or later come face to face with dynamics that, left unchallenged, can threaten people's lives and sometimes, hasten their deaths.

Some of the ways in which people's lives are threatened are subtle and indirect, such as when a person cannot afford preventive medical care or medical insurance. People who are on drugs for years on end (including some prescription drugs) often die earlier than they might have. These and other subtle forms of hastening death, or what Dr. Wolfensberger has termed "deathmaking," are rarely recognized as being what they are because they happen over time and at a distance.[10]

Other forms of deathmaking are more direct. Prenatal discrimination against unborn babies diagnosed as having physical or mental impairments often results in "difficult choices" which in reality means tearing a handicapped baby's body apart limb by limb in the womb. Babies born with multiple impairments may be laid in a cart with a sign that says, "Do not feed." People with profound neurological impairments, including those in a "persistent vegetative state" — the medicalized version of the "vegetable" label — are starved or dehydrated to death by withdrawing their food and water. People with even mild impairments may be denied needed medical treatment, such as when babies with Down's syndrome are

---

[10] For a detailed description of deathmaking, see Wolfensberger, W. (1992). *The new genocide of handicapped and afflicted people* (rev. ed.). Syracuse, NY: Training Institute for Human Service Planning, Leadership & Change Agentry.

denied life-saving heart surgery or correction of digestive tract malformations. The harshness and violence of the street culture results in countless deaths of homeless people, many of whom have mental disorders.

The Social Role Valorization Implementation Project (SRVIP) in Massachusetts, in association with the Training Institute at Syracuse University, offers workshops that specifically deal with threats to the lives of devalued people, and how to protect devalued people from these threats.[11] I would encourage those who desire more understanding of this topic to seek out one or more of these workshops. The Citizen Advocacy movement has recognized this dangerous trend, and this issue was a major theme at the 30-Year Citizen Advocacy conference in Omaha in October 2000. A growing number of Citizen Advocacy offices have supported advocates who have been responsible for saving people's lives.

Deathmaking is a logical endpoint to social devaluation. To perceive a human being as having less value is to judge that person's life to be less valuable. If a human life is not perceived as having essential, intrinsic value, then that life can be neglected, ignored, discarded and hastened toward death. When that happens, devaluation becomes final and complete.

The Essence of Social Devaluation

Facing the dynamics of social devaluation forces us to ask ourselves what kind of world we live in. Many people prefer to think of the world as a kind, welcoming place. If only we could fix things, the thinking goes, "Life would be great for everybody." Yet there have been centuries of different ways of "fixing things" and we have as much segregation, exclusion, poverty, discrimination and oppression in the world as we ever had — arguably more.

The challenge, then, is not about fixing what is broken. The challenge is a personal moral decision about where each of us stands in

---

[11] The Social Role Valorization Implementation Project (SRVIP) is directed by Jo Massarelli, and may be reached at 74 Elm St., Worcester, MA. 01609. Phone: (508) 752-3670.

the face of social devaluation and its effects on vulnerable people. Personal engagement between people with and without disabilities provides real opportunities for individuals to act upon that moral challenge. "Moral" means making the distinction of right from wrong. It is wrong to treat anyone as less than oneself. It is right to regard *all* people as of equal value, and to act upon that belief by respecting and defending the inherent worth and dignity of every human being.

When we consider the morality of how we treat one another, we raise questions of good and evil. By evil, I mean that which opposes the good of human beings — that which is destructive to people's lives and to life itself. The question of why people with disabilities tend to be treated so badly in our culture hinges on our culture's definition of goodness, and also, our understanding of human cruelty — "man's inhumanity to man." Cruelty implies a conscious intention to hurt others, but I speak here of a cruelty that wears the face of indifference, with eyes that perceive devalued people as not like "us."

In nature, the wolf attacks the weak sheep — the sheep that cannot run so fast. The metaphor of the wolf attacking the weak sheep is a powerful representation of how social devaluation preys upon vulnerable people. The segregation, isolation, rejection and dehumanization described in this chapter speak to a systematic pattern of hurtful forces that vulnerable people are subjected to over and over again. Once one honestly confronts this reality, one must ask what kind of dynamic is driving these forces. Dehumanizing forces in our culture, in our service systems, and in human hearts, are evil. I do not know of another word that says it more clearly.

Freely-chosen relationships have great significance for people with disabilities, as they do for anyone. When a family member, neighbor, friend, church member, co-worker, is committed to a person with a disability, life tends to go better for that person. The presence of someone willing to look at the world through the eyes of a person with a disability and who will act from that person's perspective can influence what kind of life that a person will have. Sometimes, the presence of an ally is the difference between whether a person lives or dies, such as when a devalued person who is highly vulnerable is in a hospital or nursing home.

We have discovered through our work in Citizen Advocacy that there *are* people in our community who can and will strive to make a difference through a personal, committed alliance with a person wounded by social devaluation. There are people who, given the opportunity, will use their common sense, get involved, and share their lives.

I do not imagine an utopian world where life is comfortable and good for everyone, but promoting voluntary commitments between people with and without disabilities is one way of helping people find hope and meaning in their lives. On their own initiative, or through Citizen Advocacy and similar relationship-making enterprises, ordinary people from all walks of life have refused to allow the world to convince them that some people are less valuable than others. Through Citizen Advocacy, people around the world have made personal commitments to their fellow human beings with disabilities and have discovered that "they" are *us*.

CHAPTER FIVE

The Perfect Gift:
The Story of Greg and Bob

Greg and Bob are from Winnipeg, Canada, and they are the best of friends. However, their early lives were worlds apart. Greg Tonn had the kind of life as a child that most people would want and expect. Bob Malo, growing up in a large orphanage, had a childhood that no one wants or expects. Bob wrote about his early life experiences in his (unpublished) autobiography entitled, "Shattered Dreams, Broken Promises." Here is an excerpt:

When I was a very young boy being alone meant, "What did I do to my parents that made them leave me in the orphanage for so many years?" It became so depressing and lonely waiting for them to come and take me home with them. I would wait every Sunday in my best clothes, eager, happy and with great expectation, not knowing they were never coming to see me ever again. Those endless days turned into years. The tears and the loneliness were unbearable. Most of the boys would be dressed in their Sunday best for family outings and a few of the other boys and I would still wait Sundays and summer holidays to no avail. I thought my parents really loved me, but they didn't, and that hurt something awful and still does today.

Why did my mother and father abandon me? Did I do something wrong? Was I bad? Why did they make all those promises that they had no intention of keeping? I sure would like to have known the answers to these and many other questions. I wish I knew the meaning of the word "love." No one taught me the real meaning of that word. I was never given the chance to show any love my entire life. Why won't the hurt and bitterness go away like they told me it would in time? . . . Is "love" measured out in parts, some for this one and that one and none left for me? How do you tell people that you love them if they are never around? I stayed at the orphanage from the years 1943 to 1954 and had a few happy moments, but mostly sad times. The fence around the place kept me in, but my parents kept me locked out of their hearts, and out of their lives.

The wounds of abandonment, and the subsequent years of abuse and mistreatment in institutions and foster homes, are devastating experiences that Bob will likely be recovering from for the rest of his life. Yet there is much goodness and hope in Bob's life. Bob has touched the lives of people around him, especially Greg and his family, in profound ways. Greg Tonn, the advocate, tells their story:

I am 44 years old, born and raised in Winnipeg, Manitoba, Canada. I was something of an under-achiever in school, and not necessarily gifted academically. I got through life in school mostly because socially I am outgoing. Sometimes I am too passive, which affects my relationships with other people, including Bob. One thing that has helped me more recently is that I got married. My wife is an achiever and an active thinker. When I have a problem, I like to talk to people and have them listen to me. My wife is just the opposite. She needs strategies; she needs a plan to get through a problem. Being married helped me get out of my head and think more in action-oriented terms, which has helped my relationship with Bob.

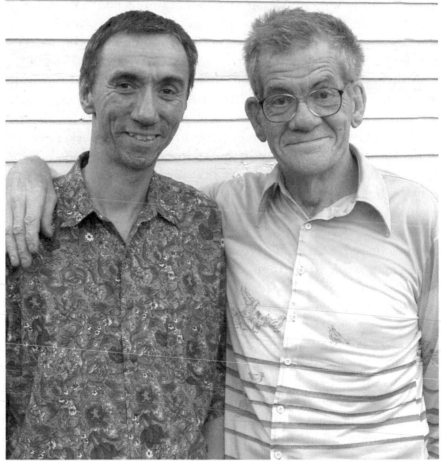

Bob and Greg

I went to the local community college and earned a business education degree. I've worked in business all of my adult life, as a purchasing agent for a publishing company, as a sales representative for a company in Alberta, and I have owned my own business for the last fifteen years. I have a passion for music and record collecting, so I started my own record store.

Around this time I was asked to join the board of Winnipeg Citizen Advocacy. Through my involvement on the board, I met Bob, the man for whom I am now an advocate, at a Citizen Advocacy function around Christmas time. Diane Slevin, the coordinator of Winnipeg Citizen Advocacy at that time, must have felt that I was the kind of person who would appreciate Bob, because she asked me if I would become his advocate. Bob does not have an obvious physical disability, but he needed people in his life. After I met Bob, I said "yes." I thought, "I can do this."

In the early days of our relationship it was awkward trying to figure each other out. Bob is articulate and expresses himself well, but at the same time he seemed distant. It took me three or four years to understand who Bob is. The things I thought Bob needed in his life were not the things that Bob thought he needed in his life, so at first he didn't respond to the things I tried to do with him.

For a long time getting together with Bob was a problem. He didn't have a phone. I got him one so that we could call each other. It used to be that I had to call him all the time, but now he will call me unsolicited. Sometimes we might see each other two or three times in a week, like when there are medical appointments or when we have family get-togethers. Or I might not see him for a month. It all depends on what's happening, what's going on in his life, and how busy I am.

Bob was born in Winnipeg in 1943. He is tall, wiry, and has red hair. He has a wonderful smile, especially when he is feeling comfortable, and he likes to talk and laugh a lot. He loves to tease people with whom he feels comfortable. When Bob was one or two years old, his mother gave him up to an orphanage. The orphanage was also a mental institution, so there were people there who had different kinds of mental problems. After some years, Bob left the institution and went into foster care. He was in a number of different foster homes where he experienced various kinds of abuse. As a result Bob is very uncomfortable when people touch him or get close to him. Even a simple thing like putting my hand on Bob's shoulder is uncomfortable for him. Any body contact feels threatening to him, as it creates a lot of fear and anxiety.

After a series of foster homes Bob found himself in a boarding home, where he was sort of adopted as a member of the household, which was the closest thing to a family he ever had. He thought of the matriarch of the household as a mother figure. She was kind to him, and he got along fairly well with the children in the family.

However, he had some bad experiences there that he wouldn't want me to share. Bob has told me things that he would not share with anyone else, which has helped me understand his emotions and how to respond to him. It has taken time for us to get to know each another and for me to understand my role in Bob's life.

Some of Bob's early experiences in life are profound. He has opened up to me about his past, about the institution, and about his parents whom he never knew. He had a lot of questions about why they gave him up, which had a tremendous impact on his self-esteem. Bob thought of the institution as a place where odd people lived, people who did not fit anywhere else and were not like other people. He thought that orphans and people with mental disabilities were seen by most people as pretty much the same and not worthy of attention.

One of the things about living in the institution and in foster care that stood out for Bob was that there was no intimacy, no closeness with anyone. He never had any visitors; and he did not know anyone outside the institution. There were never any gifts. Bob's experience of holidays was very different from most people's experience. Bob saw Thanksgiving, Easter and Christmas holidays portrayed on television, which reinforced a certain "otherness," a feeling of "I am not part of that world." He has built protective walls that hold back any emotional response to holidays, a kind of "I don't need the world. I don't need friendships or other people. I don't need their holidays." There are times, however, when Bob will talk about how difficult Christmas was. As a child in the institution he might get an anonymous toy that had nothing to do with what he wanted or who he was. It wasn't a gift given from one person to another. There was nothing personal about the experience, so his attitude towards holidays and gift giving was pretty negative. Bob never felt there was anyone in his life who cared.

Bob has a number of health issues, including epilepsy for which he takes fairly high dosages of medication. He doesn't look healthy, and he has smoked cigarettes for a long time. Everyone at the institution smoked, so it was easy to start. About a year ago Bob tried to quit smoking by using (nicotine) patches. Things didn't work out the way we hoped, and after a while I realized that Bob needed to smoke to help deal with the world around him. As much as we tried to get him to quit, smoking is just part of his life. We have tried to help him improve his diet and exercise, and we worry that the medications may be causing him to lose sensitivity in his feet, because he sometimes has problems with balance. He will be walking down the street and suddenly lose his balance and fall.

We go with Bob to his physicians from time to time. My wife is a physiotherapist by profession with a Master's in community health, so she has been a tremendous asset. She is very conscientious and thorough when it comes to understanding what some of these medications do. She challenges doctors to explain what is happening with Bob. Through her eyes I have looked at the medical system through a different lens. Sometimes physicians don't do everything for a person with a disability that they might do for someone who isn't disabled, and there is a big difference between a good doctor and a bad doctor.

Bob keeps track of how much medication he takes, and he can quote the number of milligrams of pills he has taken throughout his life. We hope that exercise and better health practices might lessen his dependence on medications. We have to be careful, though, because a couple of years ago his medications were reduced and Bob had a seizure. He didn't tell me at first because he thought I would worry. I told Bob, "I need to know. Me worrying about you is a good thing." One of my mantras with Bob has been, "I am not going anywhere. I am here. I need to know about these things. I want to be part of your life in meaningful ways, including helping you with health issues."

Bob has been very patient with me. When I got married in 1998, Bob initially saw that as a threat to our relationship. He was convinced he would never see me again. However, my wife had been a friend of mine for years, and she knew Bob would continue to be a part of my life. Now that we are married, Bob is part of our family. He is part of most of our family events, including Easter, Thanksgiving, and Christmas. My mother and brothers know him well.

Bob was very helpful prior to our wedding. During the weeks leading up to the wedding, little things needed to be done, so Bob pitched in and mowed the lawn and did some yard work — he loves being helpful. When we opened our wedding gifts, we were shocked to find a gift from Bob — two crystal wine goblets.

I know how much money Bob gets and how far it goes. With everything he has to spend money on, there's nothing left over. Buying those wine goblets was an extraordinary sacrifice. The fact that he thought he might never see me again deepened the meaning of that gift. I don't think I have ever received a better gift.

Bob and I have had good times and bad times, just like anyone in a family. One of the best times was when we traveled to Vancouver together. I used to travel to Vancouver once a year to visit with friends. One year Bob and I were having one of our sit-down conversations and I asked him, "If there was one thing you really wanted to do in your life, what would it be?" Not knowing I was planning a trip to Vancouver, he said he would like to travel, that he would like to see mountains. He had seen mountains in magazines and on television, and decided that was something he'd like to do. He had not been outside of Winnipeg for years.

I asked Bob if he would like to come with me on my trip, to which he enthusiastically responded, "Yes." It's too long to drive, that would take over 48 hours of driving time, so we flew to Vancouver, rented a car, and stayed at my friend's house. My friend has cats, and Bob, never having lived with animals before, played with those cats constantly for five or six days. He was absolutely in heaven and wanted a cat when we got back home. We took a ferry to Vancouver Island and went to an isolated forest wilderness, very pristine and beautiful. We stopped on the highway and walked along little paths and streams in the rainforest, and we walked along the beaches.

One experience that stood out was an absolutely gorgeous day in a park in Vancouver. Bob is a music lover, like I am, and we heard some opera singing nearby. We thought it was coming from a loud-speaker, so Bob and I decided to check it out. What we found was an Italian gentleman wandering around the park singing beautiful opera music to himself. We followed him for about fifteen minutes. The man was singing to himself, often with his eyes closed, very self-absorbed. Bob was enchanted by that experience. Before that opera had only been a disembodied voice coming out of a speaker. Listening to this man singing opera in the park was absolutely beautiful.

The trip to Vancouver was one of the most extraordinary times I have ever had with Bob. I took a lot of pictures — three or four rolls of film — because Bob did not have any pictures of himself at all. I thought about Bob growing up without a past, without any positive memories. Bob is a very sensitive man. Our trip was an opening-up time for Bob, and we talked about his past. He talked about how he wanted to forget the past because it was so painful. I was very aware at the time that we were creating memories. For Christmas, I framed one of the pictures and gave it to him. It is a beautiful picture of Bob sitting in a botanical garden, his hand held out smelling a flower.

When I met Bob he was living in an old neighborhood in Winnipeg that was run-down, small, poor and working class. Some homes had fallen into disrepair, and there were a lot of boarding homes. Bob lived for ten years in an apartment building through the Winnipeg Housing Authority that offers subsidized housing. Over the years the neighborhood was experiencing more and more violence. Street gangs roamed the neighborhood, with burned-out buildings and graffiti everywhere. Bob likes to go out for walks, but could never go out at night, so it was a great hindrance for him to live in an unsafe neighborhood.

We found an apartment close to my place, a couple blocks away. I live in an old neighborhood that we call the "Granola Belt," where old hippies moved in and renovated the houses. The apartment we found wasn't in a great building, but it was a great neighborhood. It was one of the few places that fit his budget, however, so there was a trade-off. The apartment Bob was getting was the same apartment the caretaker was living in, so it looked satisfactory. The caretaker was apparently moving to a different part of the building. We had seen a lot of horrible places, so we were pleased to find a decent apartment.

Bob made the commitment and I gave him the damage deposit. We got a van and I rallied a few of my friends who were quite happy to help. On moving day Bob went to get his key, but they gave him a key to a different apartment, which I thought was a mistake. We got the van loaded and drove to the apartment building. We tried the key and couldn't get into the apartment, so we knocked on the door. It was only then that we were told that the apartment had been rented to someone else. They said Bob was getting an apartment down the hall instead. So we went down the hall and knocked on the door and got someone out of bed. They were supposed to be out that day but had not packed a thing — it was clear that they were not nearly ready to move.

At that point I felt powerless. We couldn't go back to Bob's old apartment because someone else was moving in. Bob was very disappointed. We drove back to the old apartment, and in the three hours that we were gone the landlord had put Bob's furniture on the front lawn, locked the door, and told him he could not return to his apartment. Someone else was moving in in a couple of days and they were going to paint it. By this time Bob was quite upset; his stuff was on the front lawn, and we were at a loss about what to do.

One of my friends offered to put Bob's stuff in his garage, so that's what we did. This was all very traumatic for Bob. We had to take care of him and let him know that everything would be all right, and that things would work out. He was a little inconsolable, but we managed to compose ourselves just enough to get everything moved into the garage. Bob stayed with me for a few days, which was hard for him because he likes living by himself.

We learned that the building supervisor, who owns about a dozen slummy buildings in crummy neighborhoods, decided that he wanted someone else in the apartment that was promised to Bob. I think that is the way they typically treat poor people in the city. It was a lesson to me how people with disabilities are affected by autocratic people with no compassion. They are used to bossing people around and telling them where to go.

I stepped in and threatened the landlord with legal action. My friends and I wrote letters and sent copies to lawyer's offices, and the landlord responded. I don't think he was used to having anyone stand up to him. It still took three or four days to get the suite Bob was promised. Of course the apartment wasn't clean, and there were lots of repairs needed. It didn't look nearly as good as it did before. Two months later I was still fighting with them to fix the stove. This was all tremendously stressful for Bob, who just wanted to be left alone. Unfortunately, this apartment later proved not to work out. There were too many parties going on in the building, too much noise, and as Bob described, too much weirdness. So we went back to the Winnipeg Housing Authority and found a better apartment in a different neighborhood, which was unfortunate because it meant moving to an apartment further away from where I live. However, Bob now has a decent apartment in a better neighborhood, where the streets are safe and there is a nice shopping district close by.

One of the things that appeals to me about Citizen Advocacy, besides its focus on one-to-one relationships, is the idea of a lifelong relationship. Obstacles to relationships in everyday life can be difficult for anyone, and people often come in and out of our lives. This could have been true for my relationship with Bob, but I made a conscious decision to keep this relationship alive. If this relationship was going to dissolve at some point, it wasn't going to be because of my failure to be faithful.

Now Bob has people in his life who care about him and always will. Bob knows there is someone who he can count on who is not going away. He has a family that he can call on that will be there for him. He also has a role in my life, in my wife's life, and to a degree, in my extended family's life. Bob understands that he is part of something bigger. He is not just by himself anymore, and he can depend on that. All my friends know how important our relationship is, because Bob is part of my life. Walking away at this point would be like leaving my life. That is just unthinkable. It's just not going to happen, and everyone knows it. If I were to disappear, I know that one of my friends would continue to be there for Bob.

My cousin's wife and Bob get on like a house on fire. They love each other. My cousin and his wife always want to know how Bob is doing. They'll say, "When you come over, bring Bob with you, make sure he comes." My cousin's wife also smokes, so she and Bob smoke on the back porch and talk and laugh together. When we visit my family Bob feels part of what's going on. One of my cousin's children is getting married this year, and I think Bob will be invited to the wedding. I know how he is going to feel getting his own invitation, as opposed to just hearing about it through me.

One of the things that Bob likes to do is send Christmas cards. He saves up his money, buys stamps and a box of cards and sends out his cards well in advance. In recent years Bob has started to get Christmas cards back. Last year he was bubbling with enthusiasm over the number of cards he received. Bob met most of the people through our relationship, since his community is intertwined with mine.

Another benefit of our relationship is the memories. Bob and I have a history. We've had some very powerful experiences, like Vancouver, and the wedding gift. That was a very powerful thing — I can't talk about it without getting choked up. The trip to Vancouver, and the people we met, and how happy Bob was, are pretty hard to duplicate.

My relationship with Bob has allowed me to live my values. Since being involved in Citizen Advocacy I have come to understand what community means. Community has to do with informal relationships, it has to do with your neighbors, it has to do with your family, it has to do with how you respond to people, and it has to do with caring for those people who happen to be part of your community in a way that is authentic.

Although I often reflect on the sorrowful parts of life, I am not a negative person. Rather than tearing me down, reflecting on life's sorrows strengthens me. I am not comparing whatever sorrows I have had in my life with the sorrow that Bob has had in his life, but I've had enough sorrow in my life to be able to say, "What did I need when I was in a situation like that? Can I be that person for Bob?"

My relationship with Bob has allowed me to walk the talk. It has allowed me to live out my values in a way that is consistent with who I am. If I do not live up to my values, it creates guilt. I think guilt is a good thing. It can be negative, but when guilt reminds you that your actions are not living up to your values, that is a good thing. I am accountable. Being an advocate bonds your actions to your values. My relationship with Bob represents an important aspect of what my life should be. If I dig a little deeper, it goes to my spiritual roots, to my understanding of my place in the world, to my relationship to people around me, and to my relationship with God. My relationship with God influences the way I am in the world. Bob has challenged me to act in a way that is consistent with what I believe. Responding to Bob is an act of love.

Author's Comments

The gift of Bob's life, and the joy he has given to Greg and to others, cannot be put into words. The joy of Greg and his wife opening their wedding gift from Bob, the beauty of Greg and Bob walking in a park together on a gorgeous day in Vancouver, the fellowship of laughing and chatting at a family gathering, these joys stand in stark contrast to Bob's early years. The beauty of more recent experiences in Bob's life is somehow enhanced by the sorrow of his younger days. Yet these joys did not come easy in Greg and Bob's relationship. It took years for Bob's protective walls to come down, and then only in part. The barriers that Bob erected to protect his heart may have helped him survive a world without love.

Greg has grown through his relationship with Bob. He found himself standing up to a landlord threatening legal action. Helping Bob find a place to live, sharing his home, and dealing with doctors, are concrete, challenging actions for a mild-mannered person like Greg. Greg's relationship with Bob also gave other people — Greg's wife, his friends, and his family — opportunities to respond in ways that matter.

Bob benefited in practical ways by having people in his life that landlords, doctors and others have to take seriously. Bob has become part of Greg's family, and considering Bob's early life experience, what could be more important? Theirs is a friendship of fidelity, love and hope, things that Bob wanted and needed all along. Bob wrote about his hopes for his life in his autobiography:

"The things in life that I wanted most were Love, Hope and Faith. Love is having people dear to you who say they love you from the heart and really mean it. Love means giving love back without embarrassment. Love means hugging someone you love dearly and being hugged in return. It means kissing a loved one for no special reason any time of the day and being kissed in return. Love means holding your father's hand and saying "I love you Daddy." Love means having my mother near me in the good times and the bad, cuddling next to her and saying "Mother I love you dearly" and kissing her on the cheek. I wish my mother and father could have been around. I wish I could have learned as a child the difference between right and wrong and what's good for me and what isn't.

I wanted us to be a family unit in the good times as well as the bad, laughing and playing together in times of joy and crying with them in times of sorrow. I wanted to be spanked for being a bad boy and to say, "I am sorry" to them and learn from my mistakes. I wanted to be together as a family should be. I wanted to have faith in what they do each day because it is for my own good as well as theirs. I wanted to be proud of my family no matter what they do or what they may look like. I wanted to go to church together and pray to God as all families should and meet other people wherever we go. I wanted to live in harmony with each other and build a loving relationship that would last a lifetime. That is all I really and truly wanted in life, and that is what I have missed the most.

Why did things turn out this way? Will I ever find the three things I have written down — Faith, Hope and Love?"

CHAPTER SIX

"We Help Each Other Be Strong":
The Story of Louisa and Teresa

For this story, I interviewed both the advocate, Louisa Abbot, and her protégé, Teresa Ennis. Louisa is a Superior Court judge, and Teresa lives in a nursing home in Savannah. After interviewing Louisa, I had the opportunity to visit Teresa. As I entered the nursing home, I expected to find bleakness, and I found it. People in wheelchairs with blank, tired expressions lined the hall, maintenance staff with gloves and carts, the perennial TV in a sitting room with people sitting and staring. An odor of Lysol unsuccessfully covered more offensive smells. It was a lonely place.

I had met Teresa a few years prior. I thought I recognized her as she made her way down the hall, but wasn't sure. I stopped her in the hall and asked, "I'm looking for Teresa Ennis; do you know where I can find her?" "I'm Teresa," she said. "I'm a friend of Louisa's," I explained, "I thought I'd stop by to visit." A smile brightened Teresa's face. "Oh, Louisa's friend. How are you?"

I asked Teresa if we could talk, and she directed me to the lobby of the nursing home where we sat and visited. Teresa is young-looking, and her big brown eyes looked filled with worry. "I am worried about

*Louisa, she had a tough court date. I saw her on TV. I hope she's OK."
I told her I was sure that Louisa appreciated her concern. Teresa said,
"I love Louisa — she's like a mother to me."*

*The bustle of the nursing home faded into the background as I
took in Teresa, the situation, and her words. What I found most striking about Teresa was her eyes, which seemed a window to a place of
both anguish and love. I saw in her a little girl bruised by her past, trying to make it in a confusing world. Yet there was warmth in her eyes
in spite of, or maybe because of, whatever wounds she was carrying.*

*Teresa asked if I would like to see her room, so we wheeled down
the hall, and into her room near the nurse's station. I told Teresa I
was writing a book on Citizen Advocacy. She said, "A book? Are you
going to write about me and Louisa?" I said, "Would that be alright
with you?" She said, "Yes, but you'll have to talk to Louisa too. Maybe
more people will be advocates." I asked Teresa if she would tell me
about her relationship with Louisa, and she shared the following:*

Tom Kohler introduced me to Louisa. I've known Louisa
for a long time. I am what some people would call "slow." I
was in special classes. I have been here for three months. I
try to be friends with people. I try to get along and not get
upset. When I first learned that Louisa was going to be my
advocate, if I could have walked, I would have jumped up
and down like on "The Price is Right."

We go through our ups and downs. We have been through
a lot together. But everyone has good days and bad days;
you know what I'm getting at? Louisa has always been
there for me. A while back, I thought she would leave me,
but she didn't. She stuck with me.

Sometimes I'm afraid to be happy because I'm afraid the
other foot will fall. Have you ever heard that saying? Do you
know what I mean? I'm afraid that if I get too happy, the
other foot will fall.

Louisa has always been there for me. She helps me by
talking to me. A while back I thought she might leave me,

but she didn't. Louisa is a strong woman. She's helped me meet other people. She bought me these shoes. I love Louisa.

Louisa listens to me, she talks to me. She helps me. I don't know what I'd do without Louisa. We help each other be strong.

The story of Louisa and Teresa is a story of tremendous suffering, yet it is a story of hope. Louisa hopes for a day when Teresa is living in a warm, loving atmosphere with people whom she loves and by whom she is loved. In the meantime, they talk, they laugh, and sometimes, they cry. But they do these things together, and when not together, they are still united in one another's hearts. Louisa Abbot tells their story:

My name is Louisa Abbot, I am a native Georgian, and I have lived in Savannah since 1982. I came to Savannah after I finished law school, and practiced law in Savannah for most of that time. In 2000 I was appointed a judge on the Superior Court bench. My husband and I have two children, Julia, who is in elementary school, and Sam, who is in high school and is about to graduate. I suppose Sam doesn't qualify as a child anymore, but he's still my child.

I became involved in Citizen Advocacy in 1990, and was helping Tom Kohler out at the office from time to time and became involved with the Board. Tom asked me to go with him to meet a young woman named Teresa Ennis, whom they had found living in a rural nursing home in the outskirts of Savannah. He thought perhaps I could assist him in matching Teresa with an advocate.

I had been in nursing homes before, so I was used to seeing elderly people who were frail or confused in such places, but I had not been around many people with disabilities in nursing homes. When we got to the nursing home where Teresa lived, I was deeply struck by how young she was — she was only 22 years old at the time. I don't think there is anybody who isn't affected by seeing a young person in a nursing home — or at least they ought to be. Teresa was

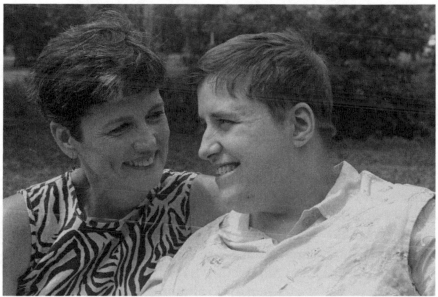

Louisa and Teresa   Photograph by Ann Curry

by far the youngest person there.

We took Teresa out to lunch, and it took some effort to help her transfer from her wheelchair to Tom's car. She and I quickly established a relationship that is a little more intimate than when people first meet, because we had to actually help pick her up and help her into the car.

For about a year I visited Teresa, wrote to her, sent her things, and I'd check in on her at the nursing home while we kept trying to find her an advocate. Then one day it dawned on me that I was her advocate. That's not how it usually happens, but after visiting her all that time, I realized that I was Teresa's advocate.

Teresa has what I guess would be considered a moderate degree of cerebral palsy. She cannot walk, and is not able to transfer herself from her wheelchair to her bed. She has some use of her arms, and she can talk — that she does very well! One of the most striking things about Teresa is her warmth. When she sees me coming down the hall, or when I walk into her room, she gives me this enormously warm reception. She will call out my name and she is very affectionate. She worries a lot about other people, and she is always concerned with how I am doing. Teresa is a loving person.

Teresa grew up in rural Georgia, and for the first few years of her life lived in an abusive home. Her mother had a severe mental disorder, and was extremely abusive to Teresa and her twin sister, who also has cerebral palsy, although to a milder degree. The twins were rescued by Family & Children's Services and put up for adoption. A good family adopted the girls, which was and is a truly bright spot in Teresa's life. Unfortunately, her adoptive mother died when Teresa was only sixteen. The twins were put into a foster home, and Teresa did not fare well there. In fact, she suffered terrible abuse in the foster home. She was shut into closets, and inflicted with all kinds of abuse. She was in the foster home until she was eighteen, and then was put into a nursing home. From that point on, she has been on a sort of odyssey, going from one substandard facility to another in South Georgia. She has moved from one place to another, in numerous nursing homes, psychiatric hospitals, and personal care homes. I think in one year, she moved at least five times. So Teresa has lived in one institution or another, including the abusive foster home, since she was sixteen.

Consequently, Teresa has not had the opportunity to develop close bonds with people. She has been limited to an institutional world, and has very few ways to distract herself from her surroundings. As a result of all that she has been through, Teresa has a very difficult struggle with depression — which would happen to anybody who had the experiences in life that she's had. Most people do not understand what Teresa is feeling or why, and people often distance themselves or push her away. One well-respected psychiatrist said to me, in anger, "She should be locked up in the chronic ward of Georgia Regional Hospital," which is the "de-centralized" mental hospital in Georgia. This was a man who as her doctor should have been her advocate, and he wanted her locked away forever.

Understandably, Teresa has an enormous fear of rejection, so she often rejects other people before they have a chance to reject her. It took me a while to recognize that. When new people, like social workers, nurses, or church people — lots and lots of church people — meet Teresa, they often form this bond with her right away but before you know it, they pull out and distance themselves. I learned that Teresa's fear of abandonment is so strong that she will test every fiber of your strength to see if you will stay connected. She worries that I will leave her, although that has never been an issue. I continually reassure her that there is nothing that is going to make me abandon her. I tell her, "You are never going to lose me." Consequently, she spends a lot of time worrying about me. She worries that she is going to make me angry, but I understand that, I completely understand that. Many, many other people have walked in and out of her life.

Teresa is extremely intuitive; she just knows things about you. You don't have to say a thing, but if there is something going on with you, she will ask and ask until you tell her what it is. She loves to laugh, and once she gets going, we can laugh continually for long periods of time; sometimes it's over the goofiest things.

Teresa, like most young people, struggles with relationships and has been very close to people who were deinstitutionalized to rural nursing homes from central institutions, many of them quite young. A number of them have died, which has been very difficult for her. Hardly anyone seems to recognize that Teresa has a legitimate, enormous grief over the losses in her life. People need to understand that her depression, her grieving, her mourning, is natural.

Over the years, there have been times when Teresa and I have been more connected than others. For example, after my father died, our relationship went into more of a dormant stage. Since Teresa has lived in various nursing homes, sometimes an hour and a half or more away, for quite a few years I was on the road with my children to visit her about every other weekend. There have been many crises, and I tended to be more involved during those times.

Recently Teresa moved back to a nursing home in Chatham County, which has helped me see her more often. I can truthfully say that there is not a day that passes that I do not think about Teresa. She is simply part of my interior life. She and I have this connection, a connection that has a certain amount of mystery to it. I love her and she loves me, but there is something more than that. Teresa and I have this connection that is something different — it is its own thing. She reminds me of my frailty as a human being. There is no one else in my life who does that. I have been a relatively powerful person, and I certainly have a powerful position, but there is something about Teresa, and about her life, that teaches me something about myself and about my own life. I would dishonor her and myself if I just walked away.

Teresa's vulnerability, and my inability to just fix things, has taught me humility. I'd like to walk in and use my motherly and my lawyerly skills to fix her life, but it is not that simple. Her vulnerability, and the pain that she has suffered because of that vulnerability, have been an extremely powerful influence on me. She has a gift of perseverance, of clinging to life, which I greatly admire. She is continually willing to put herself out there, even though that is very difficult. Being engaged in Teresa's life has been one of the greatest challenges in my life.

If you asked Teresa about me, she would be absolutely eloquent, even rhapsodic. She would bore you to tears talking about me. A former client of mine went out to visit Teresa, and she spent the entire time heaping praise upon me. She and I have been through a lot together; there have been some great times and some terrible times. In a way, she helped raise my children, especially my daughter. During the many visits my children and I had with her, we would go to restaurants and do all kinds of things, and she was constantly telling my daughter, who was just a toddler, what she needed to do, or better do, or not do. There is definitely a little bit of Teresa in my daughter!

I suppose our relationship is somewhat like a mother-daughter relationship. On occasion, she will jokingly call me "Momma," like when I get after her about taking care of herself. I pay attention to her physical condition and how well she and others are taking care of her.

There were some hard times. Whenever she moved, she was usually "dumped," kicked out, locked out, and very suddenly, I'd get a call, "We can't handle her." She usually ended up in a psychiatric facility then. I don't know what the DSM-IV [psychiatric diagnostic manual] label is for what they perceive, but sometimes she would be very ill, hallucinating, and inevitably, drugged. Things happen with her because of her deep grief, things that most people do not understand. Sometimes I would go into these psychiatric facilities, and she would be strapped into bed, terrified. During those times, I tell her, "We have been through this before, and I know what is going to happen, and I know that you are going to get better." I explain to her that there are reasons that she is feeling what she is feeling, and that is a comfort to her. Nobody else knows her history, nobody else can say to her, "Remember, this has happened before, and you will come out of this. You are going to be OK." They can't see her as a person. They don't see the person who has had ups and downs. If I am with Teresa, she's fine. Even with great difficulty, I am able to break through what's true and what isn't, because she gets very confused sometimes. When I am with her she is reassured that many of her symptoms will pass. I can walk in the room, assess what is going on, and allow her to be very frank with me and tell me what's happening. A lot of times we don't even have to address what's happened, we just move on. Within an hour, she'll be much calmer. With me, she is able to connect with who she is and get beyond her illness. We have this thing where we say, "There is this thing in your head, over there, but that is not who you are." Before you know it, that dark thing has loosened its grip on her, and she emerges.

Since Teresa has used up her lifetime federal Medicaid money, she is not eligible for private psychiatric facilities. After a stay in a psychiatric hospital, they'd send her back to the nursing home, or to another nursing home, whatever's available. Some of the places she has lived in have been hell, truly hell. In one place, every time a door opened a siren went off, and I mean a loud siren. Everyone there was lined up sideways along the walls, sitting in chairs. There were children, elderly people, people with profound mental retardation, people with schizophrenia, and people with other disabilities. Tom Kohler and I visited there together one time, and as we were leaving we both had this sense of some kind of holocaust. Not the Holocaust in Germany, I'm not saying that, but we both felt like this terrible thing was happening there. When you walked out the door into the sunshine you would never know what was happening inside. Another time when I went to see her everyone was lined up in one room together, in chairs, and they played music. The nurses occasionally did a little calisthenics, and they made them sit there from six in the morning until six in the evening, all day, every day. Teresa is used to running the halls in her wheelchair, so she hated that. She got out of there pretty quick, because she kept dialing 9-1-1 [the emergency number] and threatened suicide.

They dumped her out of there to a private home, a home where they took her social security money in return for taking care of her. However, the lady there had never taken care of anyone like Teresa before, and her husband and children had no idea of what they were doing. I went to take Teresa to a concert, and I have never seen her so drugged. I have seen her on pretty high does of Haldol, but I have never seen her like that. That night I called the doctor's service, and thank God, the next morning we were able to get her out of there. She was near death from an overdose of Haldol, and it wasn't her fault, because she couldn't open the pill bottle.

For a long time, I would say four or five months, I lived in stark terror. She was rolled out of one place to another, and I was afraid she was going to literally end up homeless on the street. There was no one else who cared, frankly, except the Citizen Advocacy office. Tom Kohler can tell you I was in an extreme state of anxiety about what she was going through.

Teresa ended up in the psychiatric unit of the local hospital for about six weeks. Then she went to a nursing home, not the one she's in now, but the one before that. She stayed there for four or five years, which is the longest time she has been in any facility. It was still a horrible place. It was unsafe, and a lot of things happened there, but for her to stay in one place consistently for that long a period, well, that's something.

I lived on the telephone when she was being moved around a lot. What I would try to do is find some ally, the director of nursing, a nurse's aide, a social worker, the doctor's receptionist, or somebody, and I found lots of allies. My approach is usually diplomacy; I don't come out of the box yelling and demanding things, I have never done that. Whether it was for my own children as a parent, or in my work, I try to use diplomacy, politeness. I would try to insinuate myself into those people's psyches, so that they would give Teresa better care, or so that they would call me in a crisis. I spent many hours on the phone, sometimes in the middle of the night. Often I was begging them not to dump her, or not to send her far away from Savannah. That would be a major impediment to my ability to protect her and have people around her. When you keep getting moved from place to place, you can never put together a community of people who can help. I spent a lot of time asking questions, and begging. I would beg the doctor to tell the nursing home that they needed to do this or do that. Many times doctors would tell me to my face that they would do something, and they might put it into the discharge summary, but then they would never talk to the people I asked them to talk to. I spent a lot of time negotiating results for her. I did a lot of grinning and joshing with people about how hard their jobs were, which is true. I tried to befriend them so that they would have some sense of "Well, this lady has been nice to me, I'll be nice to Teresa." I did a lot of things to avoid retaliation against Teresa. I'd say things like, "Teresa hasn't raised this with me, but I am really concerned about whether or not she has a bad esophageal ulcer. She could end up critically ill and she really needs to be monitored." Or it might be about bedsores, or something else. I would always have to say, "This is really a big deal for me; you'll just have to put up with me about this, but I am going to have to insist that you check these things."

Teresa is clear and vocal about what she needs, but sometimes people get ticked off by how vocal she can be. I have tried to facilitate better communications so that she won't be abused as a result of people being mad at her. I tried to help her understand that there is a line. I'd tell her, "If there is something wrong, call me, or the administration, or the ombudsman, or even 9-1-1 if necessary, but you have to know what is an emergency and what isn't." So I have done a lot of negotiating that way, too. I've preached many a sermon about treating other people the way you would want to be treated.

I have spent a lot of time talking to the people at the Citizen Advocacy office, and they have been an enormous support. I have tried to intentionally build a group of people around Teresa; I have met with groups of people in fancy boardrooms, or over breakfast, trying to get people involved in her life.

However, there have been more times than not when I have considered everything I have done to be a huge failure. Not a waste of time by any stretch of the imagination, but I felt I had failed her. My goal at the outset was for her to live in her own home, with the assistance she needed to live and participate in the community, but that hasn't happened yet. I had hoped there would be more people in her life. That was my initial goal, but it is a goal not yet realized. I still think that is, and should be, the ultimate goal.

So when I think about that, I have to back up and ask myself, "Well, what is there?" For one thing, Teresa has had very few people in her life who have stayed. She had fourteen years with her adopted family, and here we are going on eleven years now. She knows I am going to be here. In spite of her fear of rejection, she has come to believe that I will not leave her. That is a remarkable achievement for Teresa, emotionally and psychologically. She still worries about it, but my presence in her life, my simply being there, has inherent value.

As I said, Teresa is a part of my interior life. I have learned things and experienced things that I never would have if not for Teresa. Being involved with Teresa, I have gone into bedlam, places that most people have hardened themselves to or never experienced. Most people don't go there, or if they work there, they become hardened. I do not have that hardness because I am not there all the time, but I don't ever want to develop that hardness. I have seen people in situations that represent the worst of what we do to human beings. That has affected my outlook, personally and professionally. As a lawyer, I represented patients at Georgia Regional Hospital, and my experiences with Teresa had an impact on how I interacted with them. I would get a piece of paper that says the person is violent, agitated, hostile, attacked so-and-so, and I would go out and introduce myself and say, "Hi, I'm your lawyer and I am going to represent you at the hearing tomorrow," and I loved sitting there with them, getting to know this multifaceted person who had been reduced, by the experts, to just a string of sad, scary words.

My relationship with Teresa has given me an ability to be calm, to be patient, qualities I might not have developed otherwise. I try to be calm and peaceful when I am with Teresa because it gives her a sense of calmness and reliability. If I'm not feeling calm internally, she sees through that. She will say, "What's wrong? Does your back hurt? Does you head hurt?" She'll keep after me until I tell her how I'm really feeling.

Teresa has helped me understand the connections between people's life experiences and how deep and important their pain can be. I have learned how deep anguish, pain and suffering can be. I have allowed myself to face very hard, painful things. Through it all, Teresa has helped me be a stronger person. I owe that to her.

Author's Comments

Louisa's description of Teresa's life gives us only a glimpse of what Teresa has endured. Advocates who respond to suffering and injustice in people's lives must find a source of strength and surety of purpose if they are going to last. From where did Louisa summon the strength she needs so that Teresa could rely on her? In part, Louisa gets her strength from Teresa. The brightness of Teresa's smile, the warmth of her love, her willingness to reach out to the next person, are testimony to the capacity of the human spirit to endure fiery trials. Teresa and Louisa hope for a tomorrow that is better than today. Hope, sustained by love, gives both Teresa and Louisa the faith that a better tomorrow is possible, even when the practical realities and the anguish of today's sufferings seek to extinguish all hope.

Objectively, Teresa's life hasn't changed much. Subjectively, Teresa's life has been transformed. Teresa has someone she loves and by whom she is loved. Louisa offers a place in her soul for Teresa, a place where Teresa can be a real human being with a real identity with real suffering and with real reasons for her suffering. In Louisa, Teresa finds an island of sanity, a rock in the midst of a storm.

Teresa has an ally who will defend and promote a better life, better health, and better care. Louisa's stature as a lawyer, a judge and a mother, along with her personal charisma, forces people to stand up and take notice. Knowing that Louisa will come by to visit at any given time puts the workers at the nursing home on notice that they must take Teresa's daily needs seriously. Louisa's approach of diplomacy and politeness in her advocacy is firm, direct — and always with a purpose — yet Louisa knows that when she walks out of that nursing home, it is Teresa who must bear the consequences. Retaliation, whether it is based on revenge, mean-spiritedness, or devaluation, is real.

In nursing homes, boarding homes, or other such facilities where people are removed from public scrutiny, the danger of retaliatory action, or inaction, is all too present. In another instance, a citizen advocate for a woman who lived in a nursing home spoke with the nursing staff — in no uncertain terms — over their lack of response to the needs of her protégé. Some time later — after the advocate had succeeded in getting her protégé out of the nursing home — the protégé told her advocate, "Do you remember the time you yelled at the nurses? Well, they broke my finger that night." Such things happen, and Louisa knows it, and so she carefully considers this reality in her advocacy efforts.

Teresa helps Louisa discover both her strengths and weaknesses. Acting on Teresa's behalf, and facing the struggles and successes that result from those actions, gives Louisa the opportunity to ask herself, "Who am I? What do I believe? Who am I to Teresa? Can I, should I, do this? How could I not? Can I keep going? How do I keep going?" These are the kinds of questions that bring one's weaknesses, and one's strengths, to the surface. These are questions that teach the lessons of human vulnerability, questions that invite people to be good.

CHAPTER SEVEN

A Life Transformed:
The Story of Diane and Aretha

The following story teaches us that transformation of a person's life, in spite of seemingly impossible odds, can happen. Perseverance, courage and love effected changes in Aretha's life that one might not have dared predict. It is only in looking back over the span of years that one can see the life-changing, indeed life-saving, impact that this relationship had in Aretha's life, and in some ways, in Diane's life. Following is Diane and Aretha's story as told by Diane DePietro.

I am 48, live in Holyoke, Massachusetts, and am married with five children. I work full time as a nurse in a doctor's office. When I met Aretha, I was a home care nurse, and prior to that I worked in a VA [Veteran's Administration] hospital. My youngest child was four at the time, and my oldest was eighteen. Aretha, 52, lives in her own apartment in Springfield. I became involved in Aretha's life about 11 years ago after I met Len Surdyka, the coordinator of Springfield Citizen Advocacy. I was at a community meeting and after the meeting found myself riding the same elevator as Len. Len made a comment, "Boy, I would hate to be out of work [like some of the people who were at the meeting] because I love my job!"

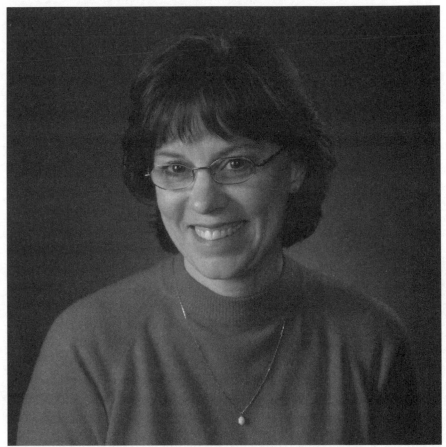

Diane

I was struck by that comment and asked Len what kind of work he did. Len briefly explained that he supported the development of relationships, not as a volunteer, but by voluntarily entering into a relationship with someone in need. I wanted to know more, so we set up an appointment to discuss it further. When I met with Len again, he presented things in such a way that it tugged at my heart. However, it is one thing to talk about becoming an advocate; it is an entirely different thing to make the commitment! Len described a woman named Aretha who had been rejected by family and friends and by anyone who tried to get close to her. She was alone in an institution. Len also mentioned that she was known to become violent at times. I remember thinking, "Now this is a challenge!"

After two months of discussing the possibility of becoming a citizen advocate for Aretha, I decided to meet her. However, Aretha was not very thrilled to meet me! She had been living in a large state psychiatric hospital for the past 10 years following the death of her baby. She was wearing nothing more than a sheet when I first met her. She had flushed her clothes down the toilet. When I met Aretha, she told me to "get lost honky!" and walked away.

Aretha lived on a locked ward. What an awful place! I was nervous when I met her, and stood way back because I heard that she had banged a heavy scale on one of the nurse's heads. This particular nurse took the incident in stride saying, "That's Aretha!" However in the ten years I have known Aretha, there has never been any violence towards me.

After the first couple of visits, Aretha was still not warming up to me, and Len offered to go with me on another visit. But, I told him, "I appreciate the help of someone coming with me to meet Aretha, but sooner or later I have to look her in the eye by myself. It might as well be now."

It took us a couple of more visits before we actually communicated. Len suggested it might help if I brought something to her. That seemed like a good idea, since that might help break the ice. I decided to bring her a pair of slippers because I thought she could use them. I went to see Aretha and gave her the slippers. She told me that she did not want them and to take them away. I said they were hers and she could do anything she wanted with them but that I was not going to take them back. As I was leaving, I looked back and noticed that she was trying on the slippers.

During my next couple visits, I thought maybe she'd like me to bring her something to eat, and I asked her, "What would you like me to bring you to eat?" She said, "Kentucky Fried Chicken. I like chocolate milkshakes, too." So that was great. The next time I went up, she was waiting for me, and she welcomed me in. I said, "How about Chinese?" She really loved food, and she wanted me to visit again. She invited me to visit any time I wanted, even to stay overnight!

I admit I had some fears going into this; the state hospital is a scary place. When I was visiting Aretha at the hospital they would unlock the door to the ward and let me in. She'd be waiting for me in a recreation room that had a TV and a pool table, and we'd visit. Sometimes our visits were very short, maybe only ten minutes, because she didn't want me to stay long. I'd sit next to her, or across from her, and try to talk. A lot of times she'd walk away, or she'd say, "Go home," or "Go away." She was very rejecting. I'd say, "OK, but I will see you next week," and then leave. I kept going. I'd always say, "OK, but I'll see you next week," even though sometimes she'd say, "I don't want to see you anymore; don't ever come back." I'd say, "OK, but I am going to call you." I'd never let go. To understand Aretha's struggle better I needed to stick with it. She did not have anyone! Unless something came up, I visited Aretha every week. I had flexible hours, and if for some reason I couldn't make it, like if one of my children was sick, I would call Aretha and tell her I couldn't make it. I tried to visit every single week because being consistent was important. I had made a commitment. My decision to make this commitment was based on my belief in the intrinsic value of every person, no matter who they are or what they have done. Everyone needs and deserves relationships that are characterized by fidelity and trust, relationships that promote faith and confidence through love. This kind of relationship is eternal.

Len told me that it would take time to develop a relationship and not to expect an immediate friendship. Len continues to offer me encouragement and support when I need someone to talk to. At times I was afraid I might never develop a relationship with Aretha. Over the coming months I helped her see that I was like her in many ways, and she became more receptive. I told her about my life, who I am, that I have a family with five children, that I work full time as a nurse, and why I wanted to have a relationship. As we found common ground and began growing together, I started to see hope for a friendship. After a while when I'd call her, she'd say, "Why don't you come by?"

After two years, Aretha was moved to the Municipal Hospital in Springfield. She was one of only nine people the state hospital did not know quite what to do with. However, after a couple of years there, Aretha moved into her own apartment with some continuing services from the mental health system. After a while I found myself speaking up for Aretha. Aretha always asked me to be at the meetings where all the hospital staff met to discuss her care. At one such meeting, I asked questions about her medications: I said, "If she was originally in here for depression, why is she on such a long list of medications? Maybe you could start to wean her off of a couple of these." As a result, now Aretha is down to about three medications.

Another time in the transition of going from a psychiatric hospital to her apartment, Aretha was not feeling well. She had to stay at a crisis center because they were closing the hospital and her apartment was not ready. Aretha was not eating; and she had severe stomach cramps and diarrhea for over a week. She told me that she was not being treated or getting any help. I spoke to the staff and described Aretha's condition, and asked them whether they had notified her doctor. They said that they had, but generally they felt that her condition was due to her being nervous about moving to her own apartment. "Are you sure? Do you really think so?" I asked. The staff replied, "Oh, she's just decompensating a little. She may be saying she wants to go back to the hospital." I said, "But these are physical ailments we are talking about and I really think you should look into it. Have you taken her blood pressure, stool cultures, even checked her temperature? She is on blood pressure medications and having lots of diarrhea, and losing fluids, could you check some of these things?" After a considerable pause, they said (in an exasperated voice), "Well, all right.'"

Aretha ended up in the hospital with very high blood sugar, and they discovered that she was diabetic. I remember thinking, "I hope that I never get like that, where someone is only a diagnosis! I hope I never become part of a system where people are numbers instead of names. I hope I can always see people as having value, with real feelings and real needs."

There was a period when Aretha did not want to see me for a long time, for about a year, and I did not know why. After visiting and knowing someone for almost 10 years, every single week, it was really a blow. It really hurt. Later I found out that Aretha had stopped taking her medications, so her blood sugars got high and she became confused, so much so, that one day she left her apartment and nobody knew where she went. Around 5:00 P.M. the police found her wandering down Interstate 91 in Connecticut, several miles away!

They brought her to the hospital in Holyoke and I went to visit her, but she did not want to see me. I called the hospital to see how she was doing. I sent her cards, but she would write on the cards, "Return to sender." She sent back all my mail, and was being very rejecting again. I think she was testing our relationship. I thought, "Well, I'll give her some time." She has always tested people. She tested the staff at the hospital to see who were the good ones and who were the bad ones; who was going to be nice to her, and who wasn't. She was always testing, so I let it go for a while.

Months went by, but she never called. Aretha left the hospital and was back in her apartment, but she still did not want to see me. I stopped sending cards, because they were all returned. I called Len and asked him, "What should I do? It's been months now." Len said, "When was the last time you called her?" I said, "A couple weeks." He said, "Why don't you just call, like nothing happened, and say, 'Hi Aretha, it's Diane, do you want to go for a ride this Saturday?' And see what she says." I thought, "Yeah, that's how she is, spontaneous." I knew that when Aretha was going through something, she might not talk to me for a few days, and then she'd call me up and say, "Hi, it's a nice day today; I think I'll go out for a walk," just like nothing happened. That's the way she worked.

So I said to Len, "OK, I'll do that. I think that's the way she would want it." It had been almost six months since I had seen her, about four months since I had sent any cards, and two or three weeks since I tried calling. After all these years, and after all we have been through, I didn't understand why this was happening. I didn't know how I was going to react if she rejected me again.

I called her as Len suggested; I was really nervous. I said, "Hi Aretha, it's Diane. Do you feel like going for a ride this afternoon?" She said, "Well, um, not really." I said, "Oh, I was hoping you would. I thought maybe we could get some ice cream or something." She said, "No." She had a boyfriend who lived in the apartment next door, so I asked if he was around. She said, "No, he's gone to a wedding." I said, "So you are there all alone? Are you sure you don't want to go for a ride?" "Well, maybe I do," she said, "Come and get me at 1:00." I said, "OK." And so I did; we went out for a ride, and it was like nothing happened. I have been seeing her almost every week since.

I tried to talk with Aretha about what happened, but she didn't want to talk about it. I told her, "I missed you. I need to know what went wrong. If I did something to hurt you or upset you, I need to know." She said, "I can't talk about it." Finally one day she said, "When I was confused and lost and ended up in the hospital, I had a dream. You were in the dream, and it was terrible." I asked her what happened in the dream. She said, "I can't talk about it."

Aretha has her quiet moments, so I do not feel the need to continuously talk all the time when we visit. She may be having moments when she is remembering something or thinking about something, and I don't want to interfere with that. She needs her space, so if she wants to be quiet with me, fine. If she wants to talk, we talk. Our relationship is really good that way. I think there are times when she doesn't want to hear a lot of stuff. There is always someone talking at her, telling her what to do. Sometimes we just ride in the car and don't say anything. Other times she will tell me things, or I'll ask her a question, and we take it from there, but it is always natural, never planned or forced.

I have learned and benefited so much from having Aretha as my friend. I have learned more about people, human nature, relationships, respect, and respecting someone's space. Aretha has enriched my life because she shows care and concern for me and for my family.

It is a miracle that she can reach out after being spiritually and emotionally battered. I might pick Aretha up and she will say, "I know you like strawberry shortcake, so I made you one." She often cooks or bakes for me before I visit. It is so humbling, because I feel like I'm not as good to her as she is to me. I mean I show up every week, but I'm not cooking all day long like she is. She really values me. I am blessed to have good people in my life, and Aretha is one of those people.

I don't know what might have happened if I had never met Aretha. Had she not had someone who cared about her, she might have gotten worse, I suppose, and probably still be on a lot of drugs. Who knows for sure, but she might not be alive right now if someone wasn't involved.

Everyone needs a real relationship. Everyone needs to be loved. To think of how things were in the beginning at the state hospital, when she was totally rejecting of everyone, and now here she is, self-sufficient, with her own apartment, and a boyfriend, making meals, giving to other people — isn't that incredible?

Author's Comments

The fears Diane had upon first meeting Aretha are understandable. The harsh environment of a state hospital and the expectations of what people are like in state hospitals — that they are "crazy" and perhaps "dangerous" — would cause almost anyone to be fearful.

Courage is not the absence of fear. Courageous people have many fears, but because they have the strength of their convictions, they are able to confront their fears and act in spite of them. Diane was motivated to overcome her fears and withstand Aretha's rejection, which made her courageous. Diane's courage was put into action by a decision. She had made a commitment, and once the commitment was made, she lived out that commitment, even in the face of repeated rejections.

Given the difficulties Diane had in establishing and maintaining a relationship with Aretha, their relationship may not have lasted without the support of a Citizen Advocacy office. One of the roles of a Citizen Advocacy coordinator is to offer practical advice and moral support to a citizen advocate. Len Surdyka offered his support and helped Diane think through practical issues. Also, Len talked about Citizen Advocacy in a fresh, "contagious" way, which helped make Diane want to become involved, and stay involved.

Diane and Aretha's story raises issues to think about when considering who will become an advocate, and about the decision process in deciding to become an advocate. Citizen advocates usually think carefully about the commitment they are making. Like Diane, they need to take their time to consider what is at stake — unless the situation calls for immediate action, such as in a crisis. Advocates who make a commitment in a rush of enthusiasm often find that they have not thought through the implications of their decision. When conflicts arise, such relationships may end or never become established in the first place. Diane understood the gravity of what it means to become a part of a vulnerable person's life, and so she took her time in deciding to become an advocate.

What makes one busy person say "yes" and another busy person say "no" to a personal engagement in the life of someone with a disability is something of a mystery. A partial answer to this mystery has to do with a person's prior life experience. Some people are more prepared than others to open themselves up to a wounded person. Diane's relationship with Aretha proves that very busy people can and will commit themselves to long-term, sometimes demanding relationships. I have found that a person who has endured suffering and hardship in his life, and who has successfully weathered that suffering, tends to be more inclined to say "yes" to becoming an advocate. Such a person is usually better equipped to see and share the suffering of another person.

Being *with someone and* doing *for someone are both important. Being with a person means being yourself, without pretense. Simply being with a person is a first necessary step towards trust. Aretha trusted Diane, which gave Diane relevant standing as a voice for Aretha. Diane participated in planning meetings where she was the only unpaid person in the room who acted purely out of love and concern for Aretha. This is not to say that people who are paid to be at such meetings are unloving or uncaring. Yet professional human serv-*

ice workers often have their own perspective as to what is in a person's best interests.

In order to retain one's role as a professional human service worker, one must have human service clients to work with. This interest can cause human service workers to (unconsciously) sabotage their own rehabilitative efforts.[12] Perceiving Aretha as a "mentally ill" person whose actions are assumed to stem from mental illness implies that she needed to have mental health workers looking after her — which validated their professional role. People defined as "mentally ill" often have everything bad that happens to them defined as part of their "illness," and yet the professional therapeutic response may have little or nothing to do with the real problem. People may be made and kept dependent by their services and then blamed for their own dependency. This is professional, systematic, largely unconscious oppression.

In the face of this oppression, a citizen like Diane enters the scene as a David taking on Goliath. Diane's conviction that Aretha is worthy of dignity and respect is the pebble that — at least this time, for this person — defeats Goliath. Diane's reflection on the intrinsic value of every human being indicates that she held high-order beliefs about human dignity. Citizen Advocacy gave her an opportunity to act on that belief.

Acting on one's beliefs is no guarantee that things will turn out right. Diane had no way of knowing whether or not Aretha wanted a relationship, or that the relationship would last. Diane did what she believed was right, and for Aretha, many right things came about. However, whether or not good things happen, making a commitment, being consistent, establishing trust, asking questions, and sharing oneself as a person, are inherently valid acts.

---

[12] McKnight, J. (1995). The professional problem. In *The Careless Society: Community and Its Counterfeits*. New York: Basic Books. pp.16-25.

CHAPTER EIGHT

History and Background
of Citizen Advocacy

Two are better than one . . . If the one falls, the other will lift up his companion.
Woe to the solitary man! For if he should fall, he has no one to lift him up.

Ecc. 4: 9; 12.

Citizen Advocacy was developed because bad things are done to devalued people. Often these things happen at the hands of human services, but as I described in Chapter 4, families, neighbors and communities can also hurt devalued people in countless ways. Citizen Advocacy was thus conceived as a means to protect and defend the interests and well-being of devalued people, and to help individual devalued persons have better, safer, more fulfilled lives. This chapter describes the historical context of Citizen Advocacy, explains some key Citizen Advocacy concepts, and is oriented to those who are interested in understanding how Citizen Advocacy was designed and developed.

An Historical Perspective On Citizen Advocacy

The first Citizen Advocacy program was founded in 1970 in Lincoln, Nebraska. Since then, Citizen Advocacy has grown to become an international movement of over 100 Citizen Advocacy programs around the world (as of this writing), including the United States, Australia, Canada and the United Kingdom.

In the 1970s, the parent movement in the field of mental retardation was at its peak, vigorously and effectively advocating for systems change on behalf of their children. Parents were fed up with sending their adult children to makeshift programs in church basements only to have their days wasted with boredom and inactivity. Exposés of snake pit institutions in the 1960s and 1970s sounded the alarm for parents to demand systems change, and Associations for Retarded Citizens (ARCs) forced states to devise community programs as an alternative to institutional placement. The deinstitutionalization movement of the 1970s and 1980s was a powerful force for systems change. Wolfensberger's concept of normalization[13] (later reconceptualized as Social Role Valorization[14]) served as a guiding light for crafting social policy and program design for bringing people back to their home communities. Using normalization principles, many programs helped people experience the kind of life — at least to some degree — that most people take for granted.

At the root of these reform efforts was a desire by parents and families to ensure a better life for their mentally retarded family member. Parents of retarded children often anguish over the question, "What will happen to my child when I die?" This question motivated many parents to advocate for systems change in hopes that a reformed service delivery system would be in place after they are gone. Since the 1980s, families have begun to realize that the brick and mortar community service programs that parent activists had worked so hard to establish still could not assure that their children will have a good, fulfilling life. Turn-over in staff,

---

[13] Wolfensberger, W. (1972). *The principle of normalization in human services.* Toronto: National Institute on Mental Retardation.

[14] Wolfensberger, W. (1992). *A brief introduction to Social Role Valorization as a high-order concept for structuring human services* (rev. ed.). Syracuse, NY: Training Institute for Human Service Planning, Leadership and Change Agentry (Syracuse University).

neglect and abuse, overuse of psychoactive drugs, and the arrogance of many inept service-providers have made some reformers realize that many of the services they fought so hard to establish were little different, and were sometimes worse, than the institutions. Intractable problems in many community programs have made it clear that parents cannot rely on human service agencies to provide a truly integrated life, or even decent living conditions, when they are no longer around to speak up for their children.

In spite of all the successes in systems change, parents and families still have to ask themselves "What (or who) can we count on?" In spite of the social reforms and many advances in human services, this question remains unanswered. Dr. Wolfensberger wrote an historical reflection on the beginnings of Citizen Advocacy:

> Let me step back historically for a moment. Initially, Citizen Advocacy had its birth when the United Cerebral Palsy Association, after years of concern, held a nationwide conference in the United States in which several groups and about 25 persons were involved (United Cerebral Palsy Associations, 1966).[15] The key question at this conference was, "What will happen to my child when I'm gone?" It is in response to this concern at that conference that Citizen Advocacy was first formulated in a somewhat primitive version. "What will happen to my child when I'm gone?" was the key initial question.
>
> Sometimes, a movement or service has a beginning because of one reason, but ends up accomplishing something else. That is not necessarily a bad thing. But we do still have the above question before us; it is a legitimate question for any parent with a severely impaired child: What will happen to my child when I'm gone? I tell parents that there is no really adequate answer, and never will be. Intrinsically, there never can be, because human affairs are

---

[15] United Cerebral Palsy Association. (1966). *Proceedings of the Conference on Protective Supervision and Services for the Handicapped.* New Kensington, Pennsylvania, November 15-17, 1966. New York: UCPA.

too transient; because of the human condition, you cannot guarantee that something bad is not going to happen after you are dead. You cannot guarantee that when you are dead and gone, everything you want will come true, that there will not be some kind of tragedy, that the world will not blow up. You cannot even guarantee well-being for a competent, well-adjusted, healthy child, because even for the most fortunate person in life, this world may fall apart. All you can do — and this you can do — is to apply a "decision theory" framework whereby you maximize possibilities for some outcomes and minimize possibilities for others. That is all anybody can ask for, that is all anybody can do, that is what we should be doing, and that is what Citizen Advocacy was intended to do when faced with the question, "What happens to my child after I'm gone?"[16]

Initially, Citizen Advocacy programs were developed to recruit and support advocates for people with mental retardation. Wolfensberger presented his seminal ideas on Citizen Advocacy to people in the mental health field, but his ideas were not well received. However, a number of key people in the parent movement and others in the field of mental retardation enthusiastically took up the concept of Citizen Advocacy, and a pilot program was established in Lincoln, Nebraska in the early 1970s, sponsored by the Lincoln ARC. The people associated with the first Citizen Advocacy program published a book,[17] and Citizen Advocacy quickly took hold in dozens of ARC chapters across the country. Wolfensberger hoped that Citizen Advocacy would also have a positive influence for change in human services in the field of mental retardation,

---

[16] Note by Wolf Wolfensberger in the archive files on Citizen Advocacy at the Training Institute on Human Service Planning, Leadership and Change Agentry at Syracuse University.

[17] Wolfensberger, W., & Zauha, H. (1973). *Citizen Advocacy and protective services for the impaired and handicapped.* Toronto: National Institute on Mental Retardation.

especially within the advocacy movement. He envisioned Citizen Advocacy as one critical component of an overall comprehensive schema of protection and advocacy that would afford personal, individualized protection and advocacy for devalued people.[18] Wolfensberger hoped that Citizen Advocacy would provide renewal within the advocacy culture by engaging ordinary citizens in the lives of devalued people who received human services. He envisioned Citizen Advocacy programs as a component of local advocacy organizations housed within ARCs or other similar voluntary associations, where Citizen Advocacy could have a positive, renewing influence through its voluntary nature and personal connection to devalued people.

To a limited extent, and for a period of time, this vision was realized in the field of mental retardation. Citizen Advocacy did have some positive influence on personalizing human services in some locales. Citizen Advocacy helped people see what the lives of devalued people are really like through relationships that were "up close and personal." This was especially significant when key people in influential positions at state and national levels had some affiliation with the Citizen Advocacy movement. However, this benefit seems to have been short-lived. Most of the ARCs that had housed Citizen Advocacy programs got into the business of service provision, and consequently, the money tied to service provision began to compromise the voluntary advocacy movement. The old adage, "don't bite the hand that feeds you," weakened the ability of service-providing organizations to advocate against powerful money-providing bureaucracies. This conflict of interest watered down if not eliminated the vigor of advocacy in all its forms, including Citizen Advocacy programs operated by ARCs. Most Citizen Advocacy programs became more focused on "lighter" relationships that did not demand much from an advocate. Often there was very little advocacy happening. With such light fare to sustain its advocacy focus, most Citizen Advocacy programs that had sprung up

---

[18] See Wolfensberger, W. (1977). *A balanced multi-component advocacy and protection schema*. Toronto, ON: Canadian Association for the Mentally Retarded.

almost overnight in the 1970s and early 1980s evaporated.

A few US programs, most notably those in Georgia and Nebraska, did not align themselves exclusively with the parent movement (though many parents were still involved), and were instead housed within statewide protection and advocacy organizations. The framers of the Citizen Advocacy networks in those states were careful to implement Citizen Advocacy with a clear focus on advocacy, incorporating the key principles of Citizen Advocacy as outlined by John O'Brien and Wolf Wolfensberger in an evaluation instrument called *Citizen Advocacy Program Evaluation* (CAPE).[19] Georgia and Nebraska developed statewide networks of several Citizen Advocacy programs, and were rigorous and methodical in creating a culture of learning and renewal through training and evaluation. Canada also developed a network of Citizen Advocacy programs across its provinces, and a body of knowledge regarding sound Citizen Advocacy practice evolved in North America during the late 1970s and 1980s. Citizen Advocacy programs began to form in other parts of the world, especially in Australia and the United Kingdom. The growth of Citizen Advocacy roughly corresponded with the spread of normalization (now Social Role Valorization) training in North America, England and Australia, as the principles of normalization provided foundational concepts that influenced the formation of Citizen Advocacy.

At the heart of carefully designed Citizen Advocacy programs was, and is, a clear understanding of the dynamics of social devaluation. Perhaps the single most important contribution of Wolfensberger and his colleagues is a highly developed understanding of the nature of social devaluation and its impact on devalued people. Wolfensberger recognized the limitations of the human service system's ability to ensure good lives for people, and

---

[19] O'Brien, J., & Wolfensberger, W. (1979). *Standards for citizen advocacy program evaluation (CAPE)*. Toronto, ON: Canadian Association for the Mentally Retarded. O'Brien, J., & Wolfensberger, W. (1988). *CAPE: Standards for citizen advocacy program evaluation* (Syracuse Test Edition), Syracuse, NY: Training Institute for Human Service Planning, Leadership & Change Agentry.

the fact that most human services embodied and transacted social devaluation. While public funds could be allocated to hire staff, rent or purchase family style homes, put people to work, and provide other community supports, Wolfensberger and his colleagues observed that many devalued people were still leading lonely, segregated lives. A major consequence of this segregation was the absence of natural, freely-given relationships in the lives of many devalued people. Citizen Advocacy is an organized strategy to respond, even if only in part, to this reality.

What Citizen Advocacy Is Not

To understand what Citizen Advocacy is, it helps to understand what it is not. Citizen Advocacy is often confused with conventional human services or volunteer agencies that serve people with disabilities. Citizen Advocacy is different from conventional human services in that it invites citizens to become advocates in voluntary one-to-one relationships, rather than to assume responsibility for several or perhaps many people as paid professionals. In contrast to the conventional approach of hiring professionals to work with people in return for compensation, Citizen Advocacy asks citizens to advocate for a person's interests through freely-given and freely-chosen relationship commitments. Another key difference between Citizen Advocacy and conventional human services is that citizen advocates are independent of, but supported by, the Citizen Advocacy office itself. Citizen advocates do not work for, nor are they beholden to, the Citizen Advocacy office.

Many people, including myself at one time, take the differences between Citizen Advocacy and conventional human service to mean that Citizen Advocacy is morally superior. In this view, the human service system is seen as the "evil empire," and citizen advocates as the knights in shining armor who rescue victims of human service oppression. It is true that many people who rely on human services are in fact oppressed. People for whom Citizen Advocacy programs recruit advocates have often endured great harm at the hands of human service providers. Yet Citizen Advocacy programs have no claim to perfection. Advocates can come and go in people's lives just like human service workers, and citizen advocates may have as many false assumptions and stereotypes about people with disabilities as anyone else. These shortcomings are not a function of the Citizen Advocacy model itself, but are part and parcel of the universal limitations of human beings and the culture in which we live.

Some human service programs genuinely meet important needs of people with disabilities. These tend to be operated by highly conscious and principled individuals who strive to address the relevant needs of the people they serve with a positive vision. They are aware of the limitations of formal human services, and they try to safeguard the quality of the services they provide. However these programs tend to be few and far between, and generally, small-scale. While most human services do offer some benefits to the people they serve, these benefits tend to be outweighed by segregation, congregation (lumping people together), and portraying people as so different that their lives must be lived outside of the mainstream of community life.

After what I have said about human services, it would be easier to declare that Citizen Advocacy is not a human service. It would also be dishonest. Citizen Advocacy is an organized approach to engaging citizens in the lives of devalued people, and most people would consider that a form of human service. A crucial difference between Citizen Advocacy and conventional human services lies in the identity of advocates not as professionals and paid human service workers, but as personal allies and fellow citizens.

Definition of Citizen Advocacy

In 1990, a group of seasoned Citizen Advocacy leaders met in Lincoln, Nebraska and came to consensus on the following definition of Citizen Advocacy:

> "Citizen Advocacy is a means to promote, protect, and defend the welfare and interests of, and justice for, persons who are impaired in competence, or diminished in status, or seriously physically or socially isolated, through one-to-one

(or near one-to-one) unpaid voluntary commitments made to them by people of relevant competencies. Citizen advocates strive to represent the interests of a person as if they were the advocate's own; therefore, the advocates must be sufficiently free from conflicts of interest. Citizen advocates are supported, and usually recruited, by a Citizen Advocacy office with paid staff that is funded and governed so as to be essentially free from conflicts of interest. In consultation with this Citizen Advocacy office, advocates choose from among a wide range of functions and roles. Some of these commitments may last for life."

Wolfensberger and Peters describe four core functions of a Citizen Advocacy program:

a. Identifying potential advocates and protégés.

b. Establishing "suitable" one-to-one matches between potential advocates and protégés, and especially matches that otherwise would not likely have come about.

c. Maximizing the likelihood that established matches that should endure will endure, and that those that should not endure will not endure.

d. Lending power to the advocate's promotion of the welfare and interests of the vulnerable person by means of encouragement and advice, i.e., doing things that enhance the likelihood that the advocate will act on behalf of the protégé with relevant vigor, competency and impact.[20]

Finding advocates and protégés
The primary function of a Citizen Advocacy program is to find, invite and support citizens in the community who will act as advo-

---

[20] Wolfensberger, W. and Peters, M. (2002). An Updated Sketch of the Rationales for the Existence and Independence of the Citizen Advocacy Office. *Citizen Advocacy Forum,* 12(1 & 2), p. 4-22.

cates for people with disabilities. Finding people who need advocates is not difficult, but having a solid understanding of who a potential protégé is, and what is going on in that person's life, can be challenging. Finding citizens who are prepared to make the necessary commitment as a citizen advocate calls for creative energy and effort. A Citizen Advocacy coordinator must be prepared to do extensive networking and individualized recruitment to find the right person.

Establishing suitable matches

A Citizen Advocacy coordinator must know who to match with whom, and who not to match with whom. A "suitable" match is one that fits the identity, needs and interests of the protégé and of the advocate in a way that sets the stage for a relationship that will potentially make a positive difference in the protégé's life. Matching the right advocate with the right protégé is as much art as it is science. A Citizen Advocacy coordinator, and those who support the coordinator's efforts (the Board or Management Committee), must have a great deal of discernment, experience, and prudential wisdom in order to arrange suitable matches.

Maximizing the likelihood that suitable matches will endure

Making the right match with the right person is the first step. But a Citizen Advocacy program can help foster a relationship in any number of ways so that it will last. While Citizen Advocacy sounds very simple — one person responding to another person — the real life situations and other dynamics of Citizen Advocacy relationships are almost always complex. The support of a competent and experienced Citizen Advocacy staff can therefore be instrumental in helping relationships last over time.

Lending power to the advocate's promotion of the welfare and interests of the vulnerable person by means of encouragement and advice

The function of a Citizen Advocacy program is not to "do advocacy," but to help citizens become advocates. As Tom Kohler puts it, "I cannot be a citizen advocate, but I can help you be an advocate."

Citizen Advocacy programs support the relationships they arrange, but they should not interfere with, manage, or control relationships. The support from a Citizen Advocacy office may include offering moral support, keeping in touch so as to know when support is needed, providing concrete information related to the advocate's efforts, acting as a sounding board, and pointing out possible directions and strategies that advocates may choose in the course of their relationship.

The Essence of Citizen Advocacy

Citizen Advocacy programs find people who tend to be unknown, isolated from the life of the community, whether in institutional settings or in ordinary neighborhoods. Citizen Advocacy peels back the veneer of misleading assumptions, helps a citizen look past labels and stereotypes, and says, "See, here is a person who has thoughts, feelings, hopes, dreams . . . a person who in the ways that matter most, is just like you."

There is a great deal of thinking that goes into determining whom to approach and what to say to potential advocates, but calling people to commit to another person is the essence of what Citizen Advocacy does. The complexity and subtlety of how best to approach people, invite them to make a commitment, and encourage them as they act on their commitments over time, is the work of Citizen Advocacy.

CHAPTER NINE

Beyond the Gated Community:
The Story of Malcolm and Eddie

Malcolm Mackenzie is not just any lawyer in Savannah. His law firm has a high profile, and Malcolm rubs elbows every day with professionals who might be considered, as Malcolm describes them, "above the fray." Sometimes lawyers get stereotyped in ways that might make one think that an attorney would not likely become a citizen advocate. Malcolm proves the contrary. His commitment to Eddie demonstrates that community leaders in high profile positions who want to have a personal impact in someone's life can be attracted to Citizen Advocacy. Sometimes such people feel limited by the confines of their profession and find the direct, person-to-person engagement that Citizen Advocacy involves refreshing and real. Following is Malcolm and Eddie's story as told by Malcolm Mackenzie.

I practice law in a Savannah law firm with several other lawyers, primarily as a trial lawyer. I grew up in Georgia and North Carolina, although I lived briefly in other states. My father moved around for his job, so we transferred a few times. I got most of my schooling in North Carolina and Georgia, and have been in

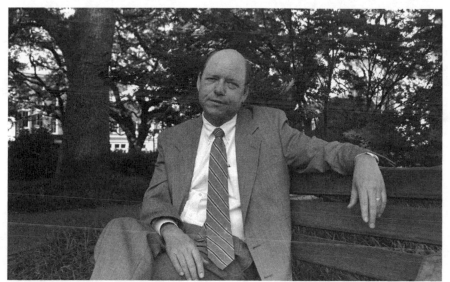

Malcolm   Photograph by Ann Curry

Savannah since 1985. I have an undergraduate degree from Georgia State University, and a law degree from Mercer University.

I was married in 1982, and my wife and I have two boys, ages sixteen and ten. My wife is a homemaker. My hobbies include reading, fishing, bird-watching, wing-shooting, bicycling, and swimming. I like to spend a lot of time outdoors, and I spend a good bit of time with my family.

I met Tom Kohler of Chatham-Savannah Citizen Advocacy at a Jaycees meeting a couple years after I came to Savannah. Tom gave a talk about Citizen Advocacy at the meeting, and it sounded very interesting. We got to know each other casually, and Tom approached me and asked me if I'd be interested in becoming an advocate for someone he knew. We discussed it, and later had lunch with Eddie. We got along pretty well, and that was the beginning of our relationship. We've known each other now for over seven years.

Eddie is in his early 30's. He has some challenges — some kind of diagnosis. He gets social security based on a mental disability, which is hard to fully appreciate because Eddie is physically capable of doing most anything someone his age is capable of doing. Lately he's become involved in bicycle touring, and he burns up bikes pretty quick. Recently he took a bike trip into west Georgia, to Columbus and back, just for something to do.

Eddie has made some choices that have made his life difficult. He occasionally gets mixed up with people who do not have his best interests at heart, and sometimes he has problems dealing with conflict. He's had scrapes with the police and other authority figures. He's homeless.

I have been called upon as a lawyer to act in my professional capacity on Eddie's behalf, but more often I view my relationship with Eddie more or less simply as a friend. I try to do things that a friend would do for any other friend. When I first met Eddie, he was living in subsidized housing, but was evicted for failing to abide by their rules. He had some conflict with the "keepers of the gate," so to speak. Eddie has lived in unsubsidized (but substandard) housing for brief intervals, where somebody had a room to let, but none of them lasted. For about a year he lived in subsidized housing that was pretty decent. It was clean, it had sufficient space, and so on, but after awhile I think Eddie got bored with the predictability of it all. Occasionally Eddie gets wanderlust and decides to go traveling. He's been to California several times, and he visits his father in New York from time to time.

The last time Eddie was in subsidized housing it seemed like a pretty good situation, but one day he decided to get up and go visit his father and gave up his apartment. He was gone for two or three months, so I put his personal belongings in storage. Then he came back to Savannah, broke, and on the street again. He now has an interesting get-up that consists of his bicycle and one of those tow-along carts that you see children hauled around in. He's got it loaded up, kind of like a Conestoga wagon, with all his gear, and on the very top of it he's got a dog box. He has a dog now as his companion. In the evening after businesses are closed, Eddie finds places in the city and parks his bike, pitches his sleeping bag, and sleeps on the street. The shelters don't allow dogs. Before [he had] the dog, Eddie often stayed in shelters, but now that he has the dog, he has decided to forego the relative comfort and safety of the shelter for the street.

It's hard to know why Eddie has taken this path in life. I don't know much about his early life or upbringing, since he doesn't talk much about his family. I have spoken with his father, who lives in Syracuse, NY, a few times on the phone. He and his father discuss legal issues from time to time, and so his father will call me with questions, generally about social security benefits. I can only assume that Eddie had a difficult childhood, and did not have the advantages that most people take for granted while growing up. Eddie has some limitations and he was in special education classes during his early schooling, and I don't think he had much support. He has lived in foster homes, and since high school, he's been on his own.

I try to give Eddie helpful advice. Eddie knows my family, and we've known him for quite a few years now. We are probably the only people he knows who have what could be characterized as a normal middle class life. I own a home; I have a wife; I have children, a dog, and a job. So I have stability. I have met several of Eddie's acquaintances over the years, and none of them meet that description. My family and I see Eddie a lot around Christmas, when most people are thinking about family and friends, home and hearth. We welcome Eddie into our home. My wife is very understanding and supportive of Eddie's situation. She lets him use the washing machine, or he'll use the phone. He comes around when he needs to, and we always give him something to eat or drink if he is hungry or thirsty. Our home is a little remote base for him.

However, we've decided that it is not a good idea for Eddie to stay overnight, unless the temperature is below freezing, and it looks like it would be a problem for his health. Staying over would just lead to problems, and I don't want to have to tell Eddie he has to leave. In some ways, Eddie has elected to live on the streets. I have given him contacts with people who could find something for him, but that would require a commitment, part of his check, and he would have to abide by some rules. Eddie is a free spirit, and right now he would rather have his freedom and the ability to do what he wants.

I have learned some important lessons through my relationship with Eddie. One thing I've gained, though I had some sense of this before, is a heightened awareness of just how disenfranchised people can be without family support. If you do not have family support, our society does very little to fill the gap. The net of our social institutions — even in a civilized society such as ours — has some wide gaps through which people fall. Some people fall pretty low, and not everybody gets caught. It is a cop-out to say, "Well, we have these various institutions that provide food stamps, subsidized housing and health care." I don't discount the need for those social institutions, but without somebody there to guide a person and act as a buffer between institutions and the individual — particularly when that person has limitations — he or she is not going to fare very well. It is disheartening to see how cut off from society a person can be when there is no family to give them support and assistance when things aren't going well.

People who do not have family ties are in a real sense disenfranchised. In a big urban area like Atlanta, it is easy to be anonymous, because there are more people. People who don't have jobs or school or some social ties can easily be overlooked. In a smaller community like Savannah, one would think there would be more interaction, but frankly, it's not much different here than in larger urban environments, unless people get *involved*.

Another benefit of knowing Eddie is Eddie himself. He can be good company, and he has a good sense of humor. Eddie gets very little respect. His problems with law enforcement, for example, are usually petty. It's not like he's robbing people or hurting anyone. Most of the time it's about where he sleeps. Eddie gets challenged a lot. If you walk around the city in a suit, hardly anyone will challenge you about anything, but Eddie often gets asked questions, or people will frequently run him off. That makes it easy for him to get into conflicts.

A lot of people view the homeless as shiftless, likely to steal, or likely to do something criminal. Somehow most people in our society have the idea that the homeless are all untrustworthy. I know Eddie, and he is trustworthy. He's developed some strategies for surviving on the street, strategies that maybe most people wouldn't look highly upon, but they are not evil practices, just practical stratagems for getting along.

There is so much more I could do for Eddie, but I feel conflicted.

Any time you try to help someone, it requires that person to want to do something. It is difficult to say how much more one could do for Eddie unless Eddie wants to do more for himself. It's hard to impose one's will on somebody. I have some roughly Christian notions about my role in Eddie's life; the basic concept of doing unto others what you would have them do unto you makes sense.

One of the reasons that Citizen Advocacy appeals to me is that it is not just a checkbook deal. It's not just, "Write us a check, and we'll take care of everything." It is a real human commitment. It's personal. It personalizes and challenges me to put into practice what I intellectually think is a good idea. Talk is cheap, but walking the walk is a great challenge.

The down side of what I have learned through my relationship with Eddie is that I've realized I am a pretty selfish individual. I reach a point where I have to say, "I have other things to do, and there is only so much I can do." I try to do the right thing by Eddie, but being a citizen advocate calls people to reach beyond their comfort level and test one's limits. We all have limits, and sometimes it is not pleasant to recognize that you are not as enlightened or as giving as you would like to be. A citizen advocate is regularly presented with opportunities to decide how far he or she will go to help somebody. I am constantly learning my limits, and testing my devotion to an idea in practice rather than just theory.

Tom gave a talk at one of the Chatham-Savannah Citizen Advocacy's annual dinners about how in our culture advertising plays such a dominant role. What really sells in advertising, he said, is "new," "improved," and "convenient." Whatever is convenient, sells. Being an advocate is not a convenient deal. Inconvenient stuff happens. You are constantly tested with just how much you are going to give to a relationship.

My parents both had relationships with people who were not in their socioeconomic condition. My mother and father had friends who they supported by making work available to them, or giving them opportunities that they didn't have. That gave me an insight as a child into how important it is to get out of the "gated community" mentality, and I don't mean the physical gated community. A lot of people live their lives "out of the fray," and see being removed from some of the more unpleasant aspects of society as a good thing. That is self-limiting. If you only look at people like you, or only talk to people like you, and that is all you know, it deprives you of a present reality. It will affect your politics, it affects how you think money and opportunities ought to be distributed, and it affects your worldview. It has an impact on who you are.

Knowing someone who is outside of their insulated world has been a valuable experience for my children. Their socioeconomic group is limited to the kind of people they deal with and know first hand, and it is good for them to interact with someone like Eddie. One of the lessons my children are learning is that not everyone gets dealt the same hand. The hand you get early in life has a great impact on who you become. I hope my children are learning that human compassion and empathy are good things. Social institutions will not always fill the gap unless somebody says, "I care."

One of the best things that Eddie has brought to my life is an opportunity for my children to see a world that would have been shut off from them if not for Eddie's presence in our lives. That is important. It is important in a way that cannot be measured by an SAT [a college entrance test] or a pass/fail. It is an important life lesson that we are not all the same, we are not all given the same opportunities. It is also important to know that you can, even if only in small ways, make a difference in someone's life.

Author's Comments

Malcolm and Eddie are an unlikely pair. The picture of Malcolm in a suit and Eddie with his "Conestoga-bicycle-wagon" having lunch together or sharing a Christmas holiday would make most people curious. Malcolm and Eddie are worlds apart, and yet they are part of each other's lives.

Malcolm's relationship with Eddie is an example of how in spite of an advocate's best efforts, the external circumstances of the person who has an advocate may sometimes not change very much. Eddie was homeless when he met Malcolm, and as of this writing, he still is.

Yet things could be worse. If not for Malcolm's help, Eddie would have no one to turn to in times of need. He might even have ended up in jail, living an even harsher life.

Malcolm's competence and social status in a sense "rub off" on Eddie, both by association and through Malcolm's actions. Malcolm's respect for Eddie as a person gives Eddie a sense of worth as a human being. In turn, without Eddie, Malcolm and his family would have missed an opportunity to see the world through a different lens. Eddie gives Malcolm the opportunity to look inside himself and examine his heart about what it means to "treat one's neighbor as oneself." In light of that kind of moral benefit, one might say that Malcolm and his family are benefiting from this relationship at least as much as Eddie is — perhaps more.

While Malcolm would make Eddie's life completely different if he could, he has learned that he cannot make Eddie live his life the way he thinks he should. Malcolm is painfully aware of his human limitations. Some of these limitations are due to Eddie's life circumstances, and some relate to Malcolm's own station in life, as he so humbly acknowledges. In spite of his selfless acts in helping Eddie, Malcolm finds his personal limits and willingness to give tested on a regular basis.

Malcolm's example as a parent extending himself on behalf of a vulnerable neighbor is a powerful testimony of a father to his children. After all the words are said, the personal action of a parent concretely reaching out to someone in need is one of the most important lessons any child can learn. Malcolm recognizes Eddie's role in the formation of his children's worldview and character. I would not be at all surprised that 20 years down the road we would find Malcolm's children engaged in helping someone through personal action, following their father's (and their mother's) example. The word "tradition" means, "to hand down." Malcolm is handing down a life-giving tradition to his children.

CHAPTER TEN

Helping Without Permission:
The Story of Elaine and Charisse

Sometimes people need an advocate most when they do not want one. Rev. Elaine Solomon did not have to ask for Charisse's permission or approval to know that Charisse needed an advocate. Charisse was about to lose her home, and her children. Rev. Solomon knew what was right to do, and that was reason enough to become involved. Following is their story as told by Rev. Elaine Solomon.

I am a minister, a widow, and I have five grown children, twelve grandchildren and eight great-grandchildren. I first came to know of Charisse about twelve years ago. I don't remember how we met, but we would see each other around town and talk from time to time. Then one day I got a call from A.J. Hildebrand, the Coordinator of One to One: Citizen Advocacy. Someone had referred me to A.J. as a possible advocate for Charisse.

Charisse was about to get evicted from her apartment for not paying her rent. She owed something like $1,000 in back rent. They were going to evict her unless someone else took charge of her money as a representative payee for her SSI benefits. So six or seven years ago I became her payee. Since then, things have been tough. I had to tell Charisse how much she had to live on each month, which wasn't much, because she had to pay the current rent plus a portion of the back rent each month. Charisse would get upset with me every month because she only had a little money left over after paying her bills. That was good in a way, because it showed her that she had to pay for her rent every month if she and her children were going to have a place to live.

It must have taken a year or more for Charisse to pay back the rent that was in arrears. I wrote everything down, what she spent on rent, gas and electric, and then I'd give her what was left. I didn't want to take total charge of her money or do all her shopping. I wanted her to do that herself, which she does pretty well. Some months she runs out of money too soon, but she's trying.

Charisse is about forty-five years old and is mentally disabled. She has two children, a boy and a girl. At the time when I first became involved, she didn't have much patience with her children. She got to the point where she was having a hard time handling them, so the family of the children's father took the children to live with them, where they are doing well. They come and visit Charisse on holidays and during the summer. I think Charisse needed the change because she was getting frustrated. It seemed like the world was caving in on her and this way the children are being cared for. She visits them and spends time with them.

Charisse is a very sweet, giving woman whom I consider a friend. She is a gentle soul that would never hurt anybody, though we have our disagreements. We talk on the phone and I try to get her to calm down when she gets upset or frustrated, or I drop by and visit.

Recently Charisse was in a relationship with a man who was abusing her and taking her money. I was upset with the housing people because they allowed her to put him on her lease. I told them this guy had no business being on the lease, and they just said, "Oh, well." He would use her, take her money, and mistreat her. It was a battle. I must have fought the housing people for six to eight months to get him off the lease and out of the apartment. She really had a rough time.

Sometimes Charisse saw me as getting in her way, especially when it came to relationships. I guess she saw me as a headache, as interfering. But that was O.K., I didn't mind that. She sometimes calls me and leaves threatening messages on my answering machine, but I don't let that bother me.

As far as the man is concerned, I'd go over to her house and let him know that I was aware of what was going on. He knew that if necessary, I would report anything he did to the police. I let him know there was someone who cared, someone looking out for her. I said that if I had to, I would go to Foodland and buy food certificates instead of giving her money. I wanted him to know that he was not fooling me. I let him know that I wasn't afraid of him. What he was doing was wrong and I let him know it.

During those times Charisse wasn't too happy that I was coming over. But I really didn't care. I told her, "One day you'll see. I can't let you do things like sell food stamps for him." I kept at it with the housing people, and finally they said, "Well, you'll have to get the guy to sign a paper to get him off the lease." We finally got him to do just that — we got him off the lease. He actually left. At the time Charisse didn't care. I guess she understood what I was trying to do. She knew I was trying to help her.

Thank God she's doing better now. In fact she called me up last week and asked me to pick her up for church this past Sunday. She's really happy. She prayed and participated. It was really nice to see her happy.

I understand why she let that man in her life. I understand the loneliness and the need for companionship. I told her that. But I also told her it has to be someone else, someone who would not abuse her, someone who cares for her. I told her sometimes it's hard to wait for the right person, but that it is better to wait for someone who is right for you rather than being content with just any man. Now she's O.K., she feels free. She feels like she's herself now, and she looks a lot better. I think she realizes that it is better to be by yourself rather than having someone who abuses you. That's what I want her to realize.

Now we talk a lot. She considers me a friend. There were times when she just wanted me out of her life. She didn't want me to be her payee. She even went to the social security office and told them she no longer wanted me. They told her, "O.K., find someone else."

She said, "No, I want my money." They told her she couldn't do that, and that she had to find another payee. Then she called me and said, "O.K., I still want you as my payee."

Charisse has family in another town, but they have lots of problems, maybe more problems than she does. It's a family that can't help one another. As far as having a solid, stable, sound person in her family, well, she doesn't have that.

I think the fact that I've stuck it out has made a difference for Charisse. I hung in there. I think she knows now that I am her friend. Now she realizes I care. Before she was just stumbling through life. Now she calls me just to talk, just to say "Hi."

Charisse has made a difference in my life. My relationship with Charisse has helped me understand that sometimes we see people and we think, "Why don't they just get it together? Why don't they just do this? Why can't they do better?" I've become more compassionate towards people with disabilities. I've learned that there are people with disabilities who need help. Charisse can't help doing some of the things she does. I've learned to accept her. I love her. I love Charisse; she is like a daughter to me.

Charisse is a lot calmer now, and when her children come they have wonderful visits. Before, she was frustrated. Now you can see her calmness, and the calmness in her children. I've been talking to Charisse about work. I think that would help her feel better about herself. She needs to get out of the house, to come out of herself and meet other people. She has a great personality and is a wonderful person. I see her as being a part of the workforce someday. I see her developing to her best, mentally and physically.

After I became Charisse's advocate she stopped drinking. Like I said, she's calmer. She buys herself nice clothes. She fixes herself up now, gets her hair done. When we go to church, she looks very nice. I compliment her.

I believe that if Charisse did not have an advocate, she probably would have ended up in a mental health facility. She definitely would not have a place to live, and her children would have had it rougher than what they already had.

Author's Comments

At the time of Rev. Solomon's interview, things were going fairly well for Charisse. Unfortunately not long after this interview, Charisse took off with the man who had been visiting her at the state hospital. Charisse went to the Social Security office and demanded that they let her become her own payee, and they gave in to her. Then Charisse and the man disappeared. From time to time Rev. Solomon heard through the grapevine what was happening with Charisse, and it was not good. There were rumors that Charisse was living out of cars and using drugs. Rev. Solomon feared that one day she would pick up a newspaper and learn that Charisse's body was found on the side of the road somewhere. Rev. Solomon talked with the local police, hoping the boyfriend might be arrested for drug dealing, which would get him out of Charisse's life, at least for a while. This went on for several months. Rev. Solomon kept putting the word out that she wanted to know if Charisse turned up. Charisse was nowhere to be found. All Rev. Solomon could do was pray and wait.

Finally, Rev. Solomon learned that Charisse was in a psychiatric state hospital. Denise Shaw and I went with Rev. Solomon to visit Charisse, who was hardly able to talk because of high dosages of psychoactive drugs. Rev. Solomon tried to impress upon Charisse that it is possible to get her life back, and that she would help her in any way she could. Charisse's "boyfriend" was also visiting her at the state hospital. Rev. Solomon was convinced that his motive for visiting was the state disability checks that would resume once Charisse left the state hospital. Rev. Solomon spoke with a caseworker about Charisse's discharge, and once Charisse got out, she helped Charisse find a place to live. The only option Rev. Solomon could find was a boarding home, but that was better than sleeping in the back of a van or on the street. Rev. Solomon has had repeated conversations with Charisse about the boyfriend's motives, and she has tried to help Charisse realize that she deserves someone who respects her as a woman and as a human being, rather than subjecting herself to the use and abuse she was getting.

Rev. Solomon's persistence with Charisse and her willingness to withstand Charisse's rejections demonstrate Rev. Solomon's loving concern. Rev. Solomon has lived through many hard things in her own life, probably more than most people. Her compassion and love for Charisse have helped her keep the long term in perspective, and to never give up hope.

Ultimately, we do not know how this story will turn out, but there is much good to celebrate in this relationship. Charisse had a number of years of an improved relationship with her children. She knows she has someone to turn to. During Charisse's better periods, she demonstrated a capacity for love and concern for Rev. Solomon. When one of Rev. Solomon's daughters died, Charisse was at the funeral as a loyal friend and greeted people at the church as they arrived for the funeral service. Time will tell how things will turn out, and not every Citizen Advocacy story has a happy ending, but we hope that the love that Rev. Solomon has for Charisse will prevail.

CHAPTER ELEVEN

From "Us and Them" to "Us": The Story of Neel and Loretta

Many Citizen Advocacy relationships begin with practical getting-things-done situations, and over time develop into heartfelt relationships. Neel moved from a place of doing good deeds as an advocate to being a genuine friend in Loretta's life, and good deeds simply became what friends do for one another. This came about as Neel reflected on who she is to Loretta, and in turn, who Loretta is to her. Rather than being regarded as a set of problems and challenges, Loretta became someone whom Neel wanted, and needed, in her life. Not all Citizen Advocacy relationships undergo such a complete transformation, but those that do have important lessons. Following is their story as told by Neel Foster.

My husband, our daughter, and I moved to Savannah in 1986. Prior to that, we lived next door to Tom Kohler's sister-in-law in Atlanta. She didn't say anything about Tom's involvement in Citizen Advocacy, she just said, "Look Tom up when you get to Savannah." So we did. It didn't take Tom long to feel us out to see if our perspective was compatible with Citizen Advocacy, and I found what

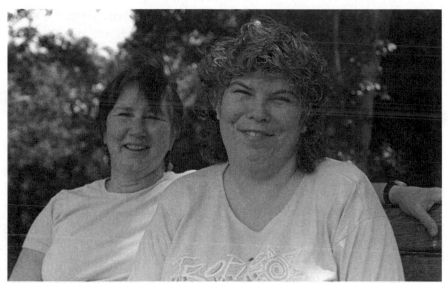

Neel and Loretta   Photograph by Ann Curry

Tom had to say very interesting. After a number of conversations with Tom, I met Loretta the September after we moved here.

Loretta was 21 when I met her, and pregnant. Tom felt that Loretta needed support in learning some mothering skills and "ordering-your-life" kinds of skills. Loretta had met the baby's father, Johnny, at a sheltered workshop where they counted nuts and bolts, and they fell in love.

For a long time, Loretta was very shy. At first I don't think she understood the difference between an advocate and a social worker. In her life, you have one caseworker for this and another caseworker for that. At first, to Loretta, I was just another caseworker, but a different kind of caseworker that she didn't have to go to an office to see. Over time she began to see the difference, probably because I'd pick her up and she'd come over to my house.

We've become closer and closer over the years, but for the first two years I was pretty much a taxi driver. Loretta asked me to take her to job interviews, and I helped her fill out the applications. I didn't realize at the time that Loretta never had the opportunity to learn how to follow up on an interview. Even though she had a high school diploma, no one had ever taken the time to help her figure out how to land and keep a job. Loretta's intentions were honest —

she truly wanted a job. While Loretta has many capabilities, she's had a hard time pulling things together in life. Some people can't ever seem to be at the right place at the right time, and life can be one crisis after another.

I went with Loretta and Johnny to childbirth classes. Their caseworker found them a place to live, and the baby was born. It was a boy, and they named him Johnny Jr., and called him "J.J." Loretta did her best as a mother. She bathed him, bundled him up in dressy clothes with cute hats and shoes, the way most new mothers do. She turned the heat up in their apartment, so the baby was plenty warm.

Then the baby developed a problem with his ability to swallow. One of the caseworkers came by and saw that the baby was sick and told Loretta she needed to get him to the hospital. He was dehydrated. What happened after that was a series of people coming in, taking the baby out of their home, and then we had to go to court to get him back under this condition or that condition. In order for Loretta to get custody, she had to be in a personal care home, but she found it difficult getting along with the personal care home workers — because they were always telling her what to do. They would get into a big fight, and Loretta would leave and end up in another personal care home. She couldn't take the baby with her because the personal care home people were in charge of the baby. As I was trying to help Loretta straighten things out through the legal system, I realized that if my baby were hospitalized, they wouldn't have taken my baby. But since Loretta was associated with all these caseworkers, and had a history with labels, they took her baby. From what I could see — and I saw her almost every day — Loretta took care of that baby the same as I took care of mine. She fed him frequently, changed his diapers, and washed him. Whatever J.J. developed was not from lack of care. Maybe Loretta didn't know what to look for, and didn't know when to be alarmed, but whenever I saw J.J. he seemed like a normal baby. It was a sad situation.

While living in one of the personal care homes, Loretta was working in a sheltered workshop. There was a woman supervisor at this particular workshop whose daughter wanted a child and couldn't have a child, and someone told her about Loretta's baby. They asked Loretta about letting someone adopt J.J., but she wasn't interested. Then they badgered her and badgered her. Finally she said she would, but she hadn't signed anything. When they came to pick J.J. up, she hadn't signed the papers, but they took him anyhow. I don't know how they could just take the baby, but because Loretta was living in a personal care home, the people in charge were responsible. Then Loretta changed her mind and said she couldn't go along with the adoption. They refused to give J.J. back to her, because by this time, Loretta had left the personal care home. So my husband and I went and got Loretta and brought her back to our house and called the police. We also went and got Johnny, the father. We took them to meet with these people, and they talked to us. They took advantage of the fact that Johnny could not handle stress. With all the pressure, he got confused and couldn't make sense out of anything. He just froze up and sat down. Then the same thing happened to Loretta. She just sat there and couldn't say anything. She didn't know what to say, and I didn't know what to say either. It was a big legal mess; these women had acted totally below board. I think they got into some hot water, because that's not the way you go about doing an adoption, badgering someone that doesn't have any representation and getting them to agree to it. The authorities put the baby into a foster home; Loretta went to live in another personal care home.

Loretta moved a couple times to different personal care homes, and then she disappeared. She didn't have a phone; I didn't know where she lived, and she wasn't calling me. I didn't know what happened. About six months passed, and then she called one day from jail. She had split up with Johnny, J.J.'s father, and J.J. was still in foster care. She spent two months in jail, although there was never a trial. Finally, she got out on probation. She wanted to see her baby, so I took her to the social worker's office to arrange for visitations. I'd pick up J.J. in my car, then pick up Loretta, and they'd come over to my house; that way they could visit without the social worker.

Then Loretta disappeared again. She had been associating with people that made me worry. One time I saw her on the street and honked my horn and rolled the window down, and she wouldn't look at me or didn't see me. She was with these two men and was holding her head down. She looked terrible, and it scared me. Then she called me from jail again. I don't know if she was caught taking food from a grocery store or if she violated her probation, but she was in jail again.

When Loretta was living in several different places (she wasn't telling me where), she'd call me to pick her up or ask me to bring her something, like food. It was a phantom kind of existence. She lived in several places, but she wasn't telling me where. Losing her baby was devastating to her; things were really bad.

One of the times when Loretta was in jail she called and asked me to call her caseworker to set up an adoption. I asked Loretta if she really understood what that meant. I told her if J.J. is adopted away, he's gone. She said that she couldn't be the kind of mother that J.J. needed right now. She was at a real low point.

The caseworker started the process for an adoption, and a mixed race couple was interested in adopting J.J., who was a mixed race child. Everybody thought that was wonderful. Johnny and Loretta both gave up their parental rights, and while they were waiting for the adoption to be finalized, Loretta got to visit J.J. a couple times. Finally the adoption was completed, and J.J. went out of Loretta's life. She often mentions him and reminds me of his birthday, December 23rd. His name isn't J.J. any more. She doesn't know the name of the people who adopted him, although she did meet them once. She said they were nice and she knew that they would take good care of him and that he would be happy. She hopes one day he'll want to come back.

Another man came into Loretta's life, a high school graduate who had been to some college. He had a good job for a while, but then he couldn't get a job. He presented himself very well, but he was a tricky guy. Loretta became pregnant, and after the baby, whom they named Joseph, was born, Social Services immediately took him away — they didn't even get to take him home from the hospital. Joseph didn't have any problems; he wasn't sick. But since Loretta had voluntarily given up J.J. — because that's what she thought she should do — they immediately took Joseph away from her. They kept Joseph in the hospital for a couple months because they didn't have a place to put him. Loretta and Joseph's father went to court and fought for custody, which they got, provided that they allow someone from the welfare system to come around and check on them, make suggestions, look in the refrigerator, watch them give Joseph a bath, and help them do certain things.

However, Joseph's father was violent and drank a lot. There were a couple times when Loretta's face was all beat up. One time she took Joseph and went around the corner to a safe shelter. So they took the baby, and we had to go through this all over again. Eventually Loretta was able to get custody of Joseph. About a year and a half after Joseph was born, Loretta had another baby, a daughter who they named Sheba. Sheba and Joseph are now doing pretty well. They have had their problems, and Sheba knows how to get Joseph in trouble, like all little sisters, but that's like a lot of children I know.

In the last few years, Loretta's life has stabilized a great deal. Loretta left the abusive husband, and now she's married to a guy named Paul who had been a neighbor. She didn't tell me about that until after it was over. It's like a mother thing; you do something before you tell your parents, because you know they are going to tell you not to do it.

Paul treats Loretta's children as if they were his own children. He hasn't been abusive, and he doesn't drink, smoke, or even eat meat. He is a clean, hard-working guy. They have stuck together through a lot of problems, and they are slowly making progress. Most people looking at their situation from the outside would probably think, "How do they do it?"

Since Loretta married Paul things have settled down for the most part, and some new people have come into their lives, primarily through their church. One of the women from the church has been particularly helpful; she gives Loretta advice and buys little outfits for Sheba. Loretta and Paul are both in the choir now, and she calls and tells me what the children did during church services. Joseph will recite something, or Paul will sing a solo, or whatever. They are really involved with their church, which has been a big factor in stabilizing their lives. They still have crises, and they have moved a lot, but things are much more stable.

When I look back on everything, I don't know how we got through it. Everything was a panic situation. It wasn't like we could see the road getting rocky and slow down and think about which way to turn. Things would happen out of the clear blue sky. Often I didn't have the details until it was too late to try to avoid the problem. We went through some tough times. There were times when I'd leave the phone off the hook because I couldn't hear it any more. It just turned to noise. Sometimes I needed time to process what I had just been through. Sometimes I would think, "Why am I in her life? Why am I doing this?" But you do it. Loretta and I have become part of each other's lives. To walk away would have been like turning your back on your sister just because she made some mistakes.

When I first became an advocate, I had this vision of helping this misunderstood woman with a different set of abilities. I had a vision of helping her make progress, with her listening to what I had to offer, following my guidelines. I learned pretty quickly that nobody is going to listen to you just because you think they should. Like most people, Loretta is strong-willed. She'll say, "uh-huh" and then do what she wants to do. Somewhere along the line I realized that changing a person is pretty much impossible. I don't know if her life is better. I do know that she is stable — she has a stable life now.

Loretta has relaxed a lot over the last five or six years. Now she depends on me in a different way, as a friend. We don't even deal with the welfare system any more. After a certain amount of time, if there's no problem, you don't have to have a caseworker. Loretta is very defensive about anybody official asking her questions. She's terrified that they are going to take her children away.

When I first approached this [becoming an advocate], it was not with the same attitude I have now. Loretta is somebody I want to know because she is worth knowing. She is funny, she is loyal, she is willing to try and learn new things, and she is a good friend. Before, I felt like I was "doing the right thing," and this was a way I could tell I was doing the right thing, by having a one-on-one relationship with somebody. You don't find that when you write a check as a charitable contribution; you can't be sure if you're really helping somebody. But I learned that it goes beyond helping people. I have learned that we are all trying to get along in life.

Loretta enjoys having me as a friend, and I enjoy having her as a friend. Citizen Advocacy should not be seen as some kind of an alternative system. That's not what it's all about. Citizen Advocacy should not be viewed as a means of "taking care of people," but as a means for people to get to know other people. My in-laws will give me things to take to the kids. My father will ask about them. Other people, like the neighbor next door, saves her son's clothes for Joseph.

Once I gave up the idea of trying to change her life, I stopped thinking, "This has got to stop. What am I doing?" I realized I was more important to her as a friend, someone she could just talk to. Having someone answer the phone was more important to her than fixing some huge problem in her life. For some people, having problems is no big deal, but having a friend is a big deal. I feel very comfortable with Loretta. The children call me Aunt Neel.

Being an advocate is not an extraordinary thing — or at least it shouldn't be. It's just being part of someone's life, and they are part of your life, rather than some odd rarified thing. It's not a goal-oriented process; it's not even a process. It is an opening up; it's including people in your life. As you get older, that's what should happen anyway, unless you're a recluse. Your life just gets bigger and bigger, and in my life, Loretta is part of the deal. It's nothing special. I have learned that everyone has different challenges in life, but everyone wants the same thing.

Through it all, Loretta realized that I was not one of 'them," I was one of "us." There are many people in the world who have a hard time getting their life together. Having problems in life is a normal thing, but some people have more problems than others. So I don't think of "them" and "us." I finally realized that there isn't any "them and us," we are all *us*. Some of *us* just have to struggle more than others. It's not "us and them," it's just us. If you think ill of somebody, you're thinking ill of yourself, because we are all part of the same humanity.

Author's Comments

Neel and Loretta's story is one of tragedy, triumph, frustration, perseverance, and hope. Losing her child struck a deep wound that Loretta will probably bear for the rest of her life. From Neel's account, Loretta lost her baby because she was one of "them." It is easier to disregard the pain and suffering of someone who is not one of "us." "They" are not thought of as people who have the same capacity for love and suffering as "us." With rare exceptions, social workers almost always regard their clients as "them." Loretta's them-ness in the minds of the people who took her baby was a barrier to understanding why Loretta's world had fallen apart after losing her child.

Neel's perseverance made a difference in Loretta's life. Yet it was not fixing things or doing things that in the end made the most important difference. Fixing things and doing things are important — there was much that needed to be fixed, and much that needed to be done. Yet Neel discovered that who she is to Loretta is more important than what she does for Loretta.

This is not to say that advocates shouldn't fix things or do things. The things Neel did were essential. Some were life-changing. Loretta became a church member, a choir member, a wife, and a member of the community. Neel would not take all the credit for these positive changes in Loretta's life, but she was present to Loretta during all these changes. Neel benefited as much from this transformation as Loretta. The following poem, written by Neel reflects this transformation.

If I Could Only Sing

by Neel Foster

Telling a good story is surely a hard thing to do. If I could only sing — I would sing one of those crying-sweating-shouting songs and that would be our story. That's what it's

like, one of those beautiful, throaty songs from your gut, one
of those songs that tears at your heart, but is a comfort at
the same time. I am humbled by the power of music. The
vibrations crack your heart open and let the story in, you
just have to be willing to put your heart out there. If I could
only sing.

I had it all backwards in the beginning . . .
    I thought I might help her . . .
    I thought she would see me as a mother.

I thought she might see herself as me,
    and be able to march forward toward the successes
    I had lined up in my brain.

Guess what? . . . Life doesn't happen in the brain!
Another shocking fact —
    everyone doesn't want to be like me!
    One well-meaning WASP can only do so much.

The first baby was beautiful without any help from me
    but he got sick and they took him away from her . . .
    because of her label.

They didn't take my baby away from me when she got
sick . . .
    because of my label.

She just needed a little advice . . . a little help . . .
    that song maybe

How many times did we go to court?
How much did I miss? . . .
    I'm not suspicious of the system . . . I'm not street
    smart.
All I could do was be there . . . I'm willing to listen.

Joseph was beautiful too, but they didn't even wait until he
got sick . . .
　　They just took him away . . .
　　because of her label.

It took two months to get Joseph home . . .
　　I knew a little more that time . . . we did it together.

Sheba was a joy . . . so tiny . . . and guess what?
　　No court this time!
　　We were on a roll!
　　Life and hope are on the inside . . .
　　Happy Birthday Sheba!!!
　　. . . I painted a picture.

I don't understand what makes some people hurt
others . . .
　　when it's too scary to stay at home you have to leave

"Home is where the heart is" . . . is corny, but true.
　　She found a new home.
　　She found a new man.
　　She made a new life.
　　The children grew — I was a skeptic,
　　but she loved me anyway — and we talked everyday.
　　She prayed for me when I didn't deserve it.

More troubles, more hardship, more worry
　　What else is new? . . .
　　This is the way it is with everyone isn't it?
　　I finally realized it.

Her man is one of my biggest heroes now
　　. . . even though we like to argue
　　we disagree about a lot of things, most things . . .
　　but we're friends.

So they're married!
   A celebration!
   A hallelujah every time I think about the ceremony . . .

The park was in bloom, and the fountain was misting,
the reverend's voice was strong; her hand was in the air,
  . . . and the flood of joy ran from my eyes . . .

I felt like hugging the world!
and we did . . . we hugged all the cousins, brothers,
sisters, children, aunts, uncles and assorted strangers.
For one moment we were all in it together . . .

We were in the same life
We shared the same heart

  . . . launched the same dream.
We were singing the same song!

Some years have passed . . .
We have some troubles . . .
We have some triumphs . . .
We choose to live in our own worlds

  . . . and they overlap . . .

we share the same life . . .
We choose to be friends.
We love each other . . .

  . . . She prays for me when I don't deserve it.

CHAPTER TWELVE

Common Themes in Citizen Advocacy
Relationships

While each Citizen Advocacy story has unique lessons, we can discern overarching themes that teach us about the value of personal commitments between people with and without disabilities, and about the impact of those commitments in people's lives. This chapter identifies 15 such themes.

Citizen Advocacy relationships cover the full range of human experience.

Citizen Advocacy relationships are human relationships; as such, they include all of the peaks and valleys of human experience.

The richness of Citizen Advocacy relationships includes sharing joyful moments, growing as individuals, discovering our interconnectedness as human beings, and finding meaning in the midst of suffering. Unfortunately, it also includes realizing the consequences of devaluing attitudes and oppressive dynamics in people's lives.

The relationships described in this book have evolved over a long time, sometimes for many years. That in itself is an important theme. Citizen advocates have asked themselves: "This person is in my life for a reason. I have something to learn, and I have something to give." When one is open in this way, the purpose and benefits of a relationship unfold, and often it is only in looking back over a number of years that the gifts of a relationship are realized.

People with disabilities have benefited in practical, significant ways.

Through the fidelity and actions of citizen advocates, sometimes a wounded person's life is miraculously transformed, including liberation from institutions. More often, the benefits to protégés are less dramatic, but no less significant. As we have heard in the stories, having batteries for her radio while living in a deplorable nursing home may have helped Teresa avoid another visit to a psychiatric emergency room. When he lost his apartment, Bob had a place to stay — with a friend who cares about him — which is immeasurably better than staying at a homeless shelter. Advocates asking questions of service providers sometimes helped solve problems that otherwise would have been unresolved, and almost certainly would have worsened. Citizen advocates have done simple things, like getting a phone for a new apartment, buying shoes, or going to a family picnic. In countless ordinary ways, citizen advocates have made a real difference in people's lives.

Citizen advocates often help vulnerable people reestablish and/or strengthen their relationships with their families.

It often happens that protégés who have been institutionalized, sometimes for many years, have lost contact with their family. Citizen advocates have been instrumental in working out conflicts with family members, and sometimes have successfully helped rekindle family relationships. An advocate from Beaver, Pennsylvania helped her protégé contact a long lost brother in California, which resulted in the brother coming to Pennsylvania a number of times to visit his sibling before he died. In another relationship, an advocate helped a man who was living in a nursing home reconcile with his son, which led to the man moving out of the nursing home to live with family.

Advocates often support family relationships directly and indirectly by assisting with practical concerns, or simply offering another perspective. There are times when an advocate encounters complex family concerns that are beyond his capacity to respond. However even in those situations, the presence of an advocate as an unbiased party outside of the family can be helpful.

The outcomes of Citizen Advocacy relationships are not always visibly apparent, but they are no less real.

The most significant outcomes of human relationships often lie beyond what the eye can see and what the ear can hear, such as loving and being loved, feeling safe, feeling a sense of worth, or knowing that you have someone to count on in a crisis. These outcomes are immeasurable. While dramatic outcomes tend to be more visible, they are not necessarily more important than less visible outcomes. Even an apparent failure in a relationship does not necessarily mean that all is lost or that nothing was accomplished. The willingness of advocates to persevere in the face of apparent failure has value in and of itself, especially to protégés.

Citizen advocates typically find it difficult to see the positive outcomes of their engagement in a person's life, especially when external circumstances have not changed much. Sometimes this comes from a self-effacing humility. Citizen advocates are not prone to pat themselves on the back or seek recognition. Yet recognizing the hidden benefits of a relationship can help sustain personal engagement and can sometimes help a relationship grow in a new direction.

Citizen advocates invariably say that they get more out of their relationship than what they give.

Most citizen advocates find satisfaction in helping others, and benefit from relationships with people with disabilities in much the same way as they do from other important relationships in their lives. Advocates meet new people, have new experiences, enjoy new opportunities, and they learn new things. Through their advocacy efforts, they may gain a greater sense of confidence about themselves and their abilities.

For many advocates, the benefits they discover come as a surprise. The most important aspects of what advocates receive involve how they are affected as individuals, which I will elaborate in the next two themes.

Citizen advocates consistently testify that being an advocate makes them a better person.

Citizen advocates often say things like, "Becoming a citizen advocate has made me a better person." Advocates have discovered sources of strength to do what needs to be done. Some have recognized their own tendencies to devalue others, and brought their unconscious assumptions to the surface. Advocates have learned to give of themselves more generously.

Wolf Wolfensberger refers to these benefits as the "engoodening" of people. While being an advocate does not necessarily make people "better," it can make them "gooder." "Better" implies that one is over and above other people. "Gooder" means that one's capacity for goodness has grown. Promoting justice in the face of injustice, or seeking another's good, are good acts in and of themselves, whether or not another person benefits. Human acts not only affect the acted upon, they also affect the actor.

In this light, being good is more essential than doing good. Being good is an internal transformation, a building of a person's character and virtue through striving to be good. To show love for a neighbor is to become more loving. A virtuous act, such as opening one's home to a stranger, or defending a person's life, or encouraging someone in despair, engoodens a person's character. As Louisa and Teresa taught us, such acts help a person to become stronger and create a greater capacity for goodness.

Personal connections with vulnerable people who need support, especially when that support is direct and personal, can "gentle" people. For example, giving someone physical, personal assistance can melt a person's defenses against the closeness such help requires. Citizen advocates have also learned the value of perseverance in the face of many obstacles. Being an advocate has given people an opportunity to live out their values with integrity. Advocates who have taken a strong stand on behalf of a devalued person are forced to examine what they truly believe, test their personal limits, and develop good qualities they never knew they had.

Citizen advocates often gain deep insight and wisdom about themselves, human nature, and the world we live in.

The stories shared in this book give us many examples of how advocates have discovered insights that have given their lives more meaning. Personal engagement in the life of a wounded person has helped citizen advocates see themselves and the world around them in a different light. Advocates have confronted harsh realities in people's lives. The most important lessons in life are not necessarily those that feel good.

Advocates have confronted the question, "What kind of world do we live in that treats people this way?" A tougher question to ask is, "What kind of person am I to have allowed such things to happen?" Even more difficult: "Have I participated in some way in the oppression and disenfranchisement of 'those people'?" These questions lead to deeper questions: "Who am I? What do I believe? Who is my neighbor? What must I do?"

Not every advocate is as reflective as these questions suggest. Whether or not those questions are explicitly raised, the lessons of personal engagement in the life of someone who is socially devalued can be transforming. Sometimes the lessons of personal engagement emerge subtly and quietly; sometimes they burst upon one's consciousness in unexpected ways.

Family, friends and neighbors of citizen advocates also benefit from Citizen Advocacy relationships.

The presence of a person who is socially devalued in a citizen advocate's life not only benefits the advocate, but also benefits other people who become involved through the advocate. This is especially true for advocates who have children. Many citizen advocates have realized how important it is for their children to have contact with devalued people, and they appreciate the positive influence such contact has on the formation of their children's character. Often the spouse and extended family of a citizen advocate will also become involved in a protégé's life. Family and friends have discovered opportunities to help in ways that matter, whether by assisting with a move to a new apartment, buying a gift on someone's birthday, stopping by the nursing home when the advocate is out of town, or just by having a friendly conversation. Sharing one's family and friends with someone who is devalued can be a powerful learning experience for everyone involved.

People from all walks of life will make serious, lasting personal commitments.

I mentioned in an earlier chapter that when Citizen Advocacy was first conceived, there were critics who predicted that ordinary citizens would not make lasting commitments. Citizen advocates have proven them wrong.

Citizen advocates include airplane pilots, mechanics, writers, musicians, educators, government workers, lawyers, waitresses, business people, shop owners, paralegals, insurance agents, retirees, investment brokers, factory workers, teachers, secretaries, reporters — people who represent a diversity of backgrounds and interests. This diversity challenges the assumption that only human service workers or family members will get involved in the life of someone with a disability. This does not mean that it is easy to find advocates, but we should never assume that only people with certain backgrounds would become advocates.

Citizen advocates have demonstrated fidelity and perseverance.

The stories in this book amply demonstrate that citizen advocates will faithfully persevere in relationships, even in the face of great difficulty. In a time and age when the social glues of community life seem to be dissolving, it is encouraging to know that people still have the capacity to make enduring commitments. Sometimes the decision to persevere with someone who is rejecting, or with someone whose life circumstances are extremely difficult, is an explicitly conscious decision. Advocates who make such commitments realize how important it is to be faithful and consistent. Other advocates grow more slowly into this realization, and after a number of years discover that they have made a lifetime commitment.

Not every Citizen Advocacy relationship lasts, nor do they always need to, but the value of having someone in one's life who will always be there, especially when a person is isolated and vulnerable, cannot be overstated.

Citizen advocates will defend and promote justice.

In the Citizen Advocacy stories, we see how advocates actively sought out what was good, right and fair on behalf of vulnerable people. Citizen advocates ask questions. When necessary, they will persuade, challenge and implore landlords, doctors, employers, nurses, aides, judges, bureaucrats, hospital officials, nursing home administrators, and service providers. Yet most citizen advocates are careful to avoid alienating people unnecessarily, because they know that generally, more is accomplished through persuasion than by confrontation. Advocates are aware that the person they are advocating for must bear the consequences of their actions — or of any failures to act.

Individual citizen advocates may not necessarily seek justice out of a highly articulated concept of justice or social change. For the most part, citizen advocates seek justice for people because they believe that the person for whom they are advocating deserves to be treated with dignity and respect.

The actions of most citizen advocates are grounded in personal knowledge of, and usually love for, the person for whom they are advocating.

To be known by somebody means someone understands you from the inside: your thoughts, your feelings, your hopes, and your dreams. People with disabilities may have few or no people who know them. It is not unusual for some devalued people to have an unknown past — their personal history lost — especially when they have lived in institutional settings or if they have lived predominantly in other human service settings. Some advocates have gone to great lengths to learn about a person's life. For a person who has been totally abandoned, the advocate may be the only person in the world who really knows who that person is.

In contrast to some forms of advocacy that tend to be based on a more procedural, legalistic framework, Citizen Advocacy is rooted in the identity of the person who needs an advocate. For a citizen advocate, understanding the protégé's needs and interests is not theoretical or abstract, but personal and concrete.

The range of personal connection in Citizen Advocacy relationships stretches from an affection and fondness to a love that can hardly be put into words. However, citizen advocates are ordinary everyday people with no more and no less capacity for love than anyone else. Citizen advocates do what they do because they put themselves in the shoes of a fellow human being, and act from that perspective.

The depth of human suffering that devalued people experience is bottomless.

While there are many benefits to Citizen Advocacy, I do not want to imply that Citizen Advocacy can by itself overcome real human suffering in people's lives. The good news is that ordinary people have demonstrated the fortitude and strength to face suffering in the lives of people they care about. Advocates have sat at the bedside in a nursing home, rushed to an emergency room in the middle of the night, and cried with someone when all that is left is tears. Sometimes all one can do is walk with the suffering person, even when, or especially when, there is little that can be done to reduce a person's suffering. There are times when the suffering, or the situation that causes it, is bigger than the advocate.

Many citizen advocates, especially those who become engaged over a long period of time, have learned a great deal about what it means to stand by, for and with a person in their suffering. Sharing a person's suffering can sometimes bring a person to insights that transform his heart. At the deepest level, such transformation is a form of conversion, a turning towards the meaning of life itself.

Citizen advocates find hope where they least expect it.

The transformation of people's hearts is a source of real hope. Susan Thomas, a long-time associate of Wolf Wolfensberger at the Training Institute at Syracuse University, once commented, "There is great hope; it's just not where we usually look for it." Citizen advocates tend to be hopeful people, though not without moments of doubt or even despair. Relationships do not last when there is no hope for a better tomorrow. Advocates are often disappointed by false hopes — hopes that a system will provide an answer, that permanence will be secured, or that a good service will solve all problems. When these hopes turn to disappointment, advocates must search elsewhere. They may find hope in the relationship itself, and are often inspired by the very person they are trying to help. In a sense, trying to make something good happen is its own source of hope. Doing the right thing in standing by, for and with someone is itself hopeful, whether or not other hopes are ever realized.

The community, and by extension, society, benefits from personal engagements between its valued and devalued members.

Personal engagement among valued and devalued members of a community broadens social tolerance of differences, and helps build a more accepting community. Tom Kohler speaks of an advocate sitting at a lunch counter with someone who is devalued as a radical act, just as sitting at a lunch counter with an African-American would have been in the American South in the 1960s. It is an act that goes against cultural norms that define some people as belonging together and other people as belonging somewhere else, or anywhere else, rather than here among "us." An advocate who takes up with someone who is marginalized and beyond the gated community counters these cultural assumptions.

Often Citizen Advocacy relationships will have unforeseen ripple effects in a community. For example, one citizen advocate told me that he hired a woman who is hearing impaired to work in his company. He said that had he never been a citizen advocate, he might not have given the woman fair consideration. His experience as an advocate inspired him to work out ways to accommodate her impairment. In recruiting an advocate for a young man who was paralyzed from a neck injury, we talked with a number of prominent businessmen in the community, one of whom became his advocate. Years later, we discovered that some of these same business people we had talked to — along with others they had recruited — had established a foundation to raise funds to assist disabled members of their community with accessible housing and transportation. The current trustees of this foundation probably have no idea how Citizen Advocacy planted the seed for this enterprise, which is part of the beauty of the ripple effect.

Most people have some influence over others with whom they have personal contact. If a local Citizen Advocacy program makes 200 matches over 20 years, each match may involve another five to ten people in one way or another. That means that over those 20 years, 1,000 to 2,000 people in that community will have direct, personal contact with a devalued person, whether over a short or extended period of time. That is true social change — direct, personal, one person at a time. On the broadest scale, the socio-political ideals of equality and justice, along with the values of love and compassion, are affirmed by examples of Citizen Advocacy relationships in tangible, practical ways.

Conclusion to the themes: The strength and vulnerability of human relationships

Citizen Advocacy is bittersweet.[21] Witnessing the depth of how people have been hurt in life, and at the same time appreciating the

---

[21] I credit Tom Kohler with this insight.

capacity of the human spirit for the fullness of life and love, is bitter and sweet. The bitterness of the pain and suffering in people's lives is matched only by the meaning that is found in sharing both joy and sorrow.

The strength of Citizen Advocacy is that it is based on human relationships. The weakness of Citizen Advocacy is ... that it is based on human relationships. We humans are fragile and weak. Our lives can be turned upside down in the blink of an eye through a personal loss or tragedy. Not only are our human frames subject to the forces of the world in which we live, we also struggle with internal limitations. We all struggle with pride and selfishness, and human existence is fraught with weakness and vulnerability. This will always be so, even when life has many joys and blessings.

In spite of our weaknesses, we do have the capacity for selfless love, sincerity of purpose, and purity of giving. The beauty and preciousness of life are found in the simplest of human acts — a smile, a warm embrace, a listening ear. Life's beauty and preciousness are also found in acts of courage and fidelity — challenging a landlord, questioning a doctor, welcoming someone into a family, and adopting a child. The stories shared in this book are examples of endurance and perseverance through many hard trials in the midst of suffering. From simple friendship to staring down the face of death, the strength of human love and integrity of virtue has shown itself in these stories of personal commitment.

People are weak and strong, selfish and beautiful, dark and light. It is in the in-between spaces that people form human relationships, for we bring both the darkest parts of ourselves and the sublime beauty of our hearts to relationships with our neighbor. When we relate to one another we hold up a mirror to ourselves, a mirror that shows us what is inside. Being present to a vulnerable person is an opportunity to see what is in the mirror. What we see of ourselves depends in part on what we see in the other person. If what we see is a human being of great worth and dignity, our own worth and dignity shine forth. If on the other hand what we see is one of "them," the mirror darkens, and the darkness of our own soul obscures the light that we fail to see in the heart of the human being whom we call disabled.

CHAPTER THIRTEEN

Some Advice and Suggestions for Advocates

Whether one becomes engaged in the life of a devalued person through a Citizen Advocacy office, through a similar relationship-making enterprise, or through one's own initiative, there are a number of lessons from Citizen Advocacy that may be helpful when engaging in such relationships. Readers who want a more thorough understanding of the rationales that underlie the suggestions that follow may want to first read Appendix A, "An Orientation to Citizen Advocacy Principles." The principles of Citizen Advocacy incorporate a number of safeguards that are helpful to citizen advocates as they assume their advocacy role and begin to engage in advocacy on behalf of a devalued person.

On establishing a relationship

In Citizen Advocacy, especially in the context of a long-term relationship, advocates are asked to step into the stream of a person's life in the present, look back upon the past, and anticipate the future. This requires spending time with a person. The amount of time varies from person to person and from situation to situation. In the beginning of a relationship, it is sometimes advisable to spend brief periods of time, though frequent and regular, to get to know a person and gently introduce oneself into a person's life. For other people, one may need to spend a great deal of time getting to know a person from the outset.

Knowing a person can take a lifetime. Even among the closest of human relationships — such as husband and wife, parent and child, brother and sister — getting to know a person is a never-ending quest. The same is true for knowing someone with a disability. Gaining a clear understanding of a person who has been rejected and hurt in life can be even more difficult and may take a long time.

Most of the Citizen Advocacy stories selected for this book are, or eventually became, mutual, trusting relationships. Yet not all relationships in Citizen Advocacy are mutual. Take, for example, an advocacy relationship with someone who is in a coma, or someone with advanced dementia. Ordinarily such relationships would not be thought of as reciprocal or mutual. Yet the fact that a person cannot communicate makes a person all the more vulnerable, which makes having an advocate all the more important. Even in these situations it is necessary to try to understand the life experience of a person who cannot or will not communicate. For instance, an advocate may develop an understanding of a person with advanced dementia by sitting at her bedside for hours, or even days, to gain a more intuitive understanding of and identification with a person.

There are times when a citizen advocate may have to step in to protect a person or to resolve a situation in a crisis or emergency, and there is no time to get to know the protégé. There may also be times when information about a person is not forthcoming, such as when an advocate is denied access to the protégé or to information about the protégé. Whenever possible, however, advocates should know a person in sufficient depth before trying to represent the interests of that person. An obvious exception to this is when the needs of a person are immediate and urgent. Still, the advocate needs to find out as much information as he or she can, and yet act in a timely way to prevent harm and protect the person in a crisis.

As the advocate's understanding of the person evolves, so too may her role evolve according to new insights about the person and his circumstances in life. A key function of a Citizen Advocacy office is to offer competent, wise support to an advocate as he or she defines her role in a protégé's life. Advocates should also be prepared for surprises — both good ones and bad ones — as life can be unpredictable, and the events that unfold in a person's life will call for flexibility and change.

On making a commitment

"I'm too busy." People often say or think these words when invited to become a citizen advocate. Some will say outright, "I'm too busy," while others say it more indirectly. Some people do have too much going on in their lives to become a citizen advocate, although that may be temporary. I tend to be busier than I would like, and when asked to do something over and above what I am doing already, I tend to shrink back, so I hardly blame people for having a similar reaction when invited to become an advocate.

Yet there is some truth to the familiar adage, "If you want something done, ask a busy person to do it." At one time I thought that people sitting at home watching soap operas with a lot of time on their hands might make good advocates. Surely Citizen Advocacy offered something more meaningful to do with their time. Yet as Denise Shaw often points out, people sitting at home watching soap operas tend to be people who are not necessarily interested in the lives of real people. In Citizen Advocacy, we look for people who are oriented towards real people, and who reach beyond themselves.

I submit that the central issue is not about time, but focus. That is, what (or who) do we focus on in our use of time? If we assume that people are more important than objects or things, it follows that who we spend time with is more important than what we spend time on. Who we spend time with might be ourselves, our families, our friends, our neighbors, our co-workers, our community. Or, we might spend all our time with movie actors, TV personalities, sports figures and the Internet.

The people who tend to make good advocates are the people who focus their time on real people. When we approach them, we ask them to include someone with a disability as one of those people. Some people are aware that they have become too preoccupied with external things and want to do something more meaningful with their time. As one advocate said, "I think becoming an advocate will help me become less self-involved." And indeed for that person, it did.

It is good for a potential advocate to reflect carefully before, during and after making a commitment to a relationship on what the nature of that commitment is or will be. A conscious commitment is more likely to last, and is more likely — though by no means guaranteed — to bear the fruit that one hopes for in becoming an advocate.

On looking at the world through the eyes of another person

I have said that it is crucial that an advocate try to look at the world from the perspective of her protégé. I repeat this because nothing is more important to a Citizen Advocacy relationship — or to any human relationship. While we can never know the whole truth of another person's life, some truths are only revealed when we see the world, and ourselves, through the eyes of another person.

Engagement in the life of someone who has been deeply wounded in life can open one's mind and heart to reality. When we see the world through another person's eyes, we can get a glimpse of truth that offers profound insight into a reality unknowable by reason alone. The essence of this reality is that every person has unique dignity and worth as a human being, a concept I explore further in the next chapter.

When advocating for someone who is not regarded by many as having inherent value, a basic foundational question an advocate must ask is, "Do I believe that this person's life is as valuable as my own?" A related question is, "Do I recognize this person as my sister or brother?"

These are challenging questions, especially when considering people who have severe physical and mental impairments. Answering these questions requires that we look beyond the physical to find the answers.

On making sacrifices for others

Most of us, whether we admit it or not, tend to put ourselves at the center of the universe and look at the world through self-colored glasses. It is possible to overcome our selfish natures, but it takes work, love and wisdom — and in my worldview, grace — to be in selfless relationship with others. The work of overcoming selfishness involves self-denial — a concept antithetical to dominant modern values. Denial of one's self is heresy to a culture that promotes self-satisfaction, self-esteem, self-fulfillment, self-actualization — rather than self-sacrifice.

It is good to invite people to make sacrifices. Most people perceive sacrifice as giving up some treasured possession, which is believed to cause unhappiness. The concept of sacrifice, however, has a deeper meaning. Sacrifice is derived from the Latin sacra, or "sacred", and fica, meaning, "to make." Sacred is a word that means, "set apart." Sacrifice, then, means to make sacred, or set apart, our time, our energy, our resources, and ourselves.

On gaining standing as an advocate

One of the benefits of becoming involved in a devalued person's life through Citizen Advocacy is that the sanction of a Citizen Advocacy office can give the advocate a relevant standing in that person's life. Good matching by a Citizen Advocacy program helps establish and clarify a role and purpose for having an advocate. However, advocates should not assume that a role suggested by the Citizen Advocacy staff is what is most relevant to a person's life and circumstances. In a relatively short time, the advocate will know the protégé far better than the Citizen Advocacy staff, and after all, it is the advocate who is making the commitment, and it is the advocate who must act. While being open to the advice and suggestions of others — especially the Citizen Advocacy staff — a citizen advocate should use his own judgment and imagination as to what kind of role makes the most sense, and how best to fulfill that role. In most instances, the person who needs an advocate, and often her family, have agreed to having an advocate and may have requested one. If there is no such agreement, as when a person cannot or will not communicate, there should be clear reasons why a person needs advocacy and protection.

More and more people are familiar with the concept of advocacy these days, and so when a citizen advocate can say, "I am so-and-so's advocate," it can open doors and help the advocate gain a foothold to say or do what needs to be said or done. Often such standing is necessary to gain access to meetings where decisions are made that will impact a protégé's life, such as human service planning meetings, doctor's appointments, medical decision-making meetings, educational planning meetings, and others.

Identifying oneself as an "advocate," however, can sometimes create problems. A lot of things get done by various people and groups in the name of advocacy in an acrimonious, adversarial, technocratic fashion, which may have little or nothing to do with the person's true interests. Saying, "I am an advocate" to people who have had negative encounters with that kind of advocacy — whether for good purposes or bad — may invite resistance and close the door to the advocate's efforts. People may become defensive, and there is often great confusion about what the role of a citizen advocate is supposed to be. Even though the concept of advocacy has become more familiar in human services, and to some extent in the broader culture, people still stumble over the spelling or pronunciation of the word "advocacy," and for the most part, their impression of advocacy is something legal, formal, and generally, distasteful.

Many people, especially those in human services, assume that Citizen Advocacy is a litigious, "give-me-what-I-want-or-I'll-sue" form of advocacy. In particular, professional service workers fear lawsuits, media releases, and threats to their reputations. On rare occasions, citizen advocates do file lawsuits, but generally speaking, they have found that the court system is not the best way to solve human problems. Sometimes a legal approach is necessary, but it tends to create more problems than it solves, as people can become quite hateful and full of revenge because of the adversarial nature of the process.

It sometimes happens that advocacy on behalf of an individual has a secondary effect that has a positive impact on a system or policy, which is fine, but a citizen advocate is focused on one person and how that person's life and circumstances can improve, rather than changing a system.

Considering all the above, citizen advocates have to judge how, when and if to use the term "advocacy" or "advocate." A citizen advocate will commonly tell human service workers, landlords, doctors, etc., that he or she is a friend of the person and/or a concerned citizen, unless the word "advocate" is necessary to get through the door. However, identifying oneself as an advocate may get people to listen. People are more likely to listen to an advocate who is recognized as a committed ally, an ally who is not here today and gone tomorrow. Gaining a relevant standing in a person's life will almost always take time, and always, commitment. There are no shortcuts to gaining the status of a committed ally other than being a committed ally, which means withstanding trials and standing the test of time.

Some tips on how to actually advocate

Let us suppose that a citizen advocate has established a relationship, knows the person for whom he or she is an advocate fairly well, tries to look at the world through that person's eyes, has made a commitment, is prepared to make sacrifices, and has relevant standing in the person's life. With these in place, a citizen advocate is ready to "represent the person's interests as if those interests were her own" through words and actions.

A citizen advocate must be willing to stand up for a devalued person. As W.W. Law, the dean of Savannah's civil rights community once put it, "Compassion and backbone — you want people with compassion and backbone."[22] Actions in the world define who we are. An advocate who speaks up for someone defines himself or herself as a person who speaks up. An advocate who takes action to defend and support someone defines himself as a defender and sup-

---

[22] W.W. Law. Personal communication with Tom Kohler, April, 2003.

porter. When these actions emerge through seeing the world through the eyes of the protégé, the advocacy relationship is personal. Citizen Advocacy is always personal in the sense that it is face-to-face, eye-to-eye, and person-to-person. Following are some suggestions for speaking up on another person's behalf. I am indebted to the teaching of Wolf Wolfensberger for many of these suggestions.

Treat people, including adversaries, with respect.

This is one of those things that should go without saying. However, speaking up for someone you care about raises understandable emotions, and in the heat of the moment, those emotions can take over and become counterproductive. In Citizen Advocacy, advocates are encouraged to be passionate as they promote justice, yet passion must be constructively directed. If one expects the person being advocated for to be treated with dignity and respect, then one needs to show that same respect for the dignity of the person on the other side of the table. This does not mean that the vigor of one's advocacy should be watered down or weakened. It is possible to be strong, passionate and respectful at the same time. Questioning or even denouncing a person's actions can be done without judging a person's motives or denouncing the person responsible for those actions.

Ask questions.

Speaking up for someone almost always means asking questions. I will not prescribe the details of what kinds of questions an advocate should ask, but I will make a few suggestions regarding the style and posture of question-asking. First, avoid making assumptions based on limited information. Ill-informed questions based on incorrect assumptions can damage the credibility of an advocate in short order. Asking questions is a fact-finding exercise. Examples of such questions are, "When has so-and-so last seen a doctor? What was he (or she) being seen or treated for?" Once one has the factual information that is needed in a given situation, then an advocate can formulate questions that are of a more challenging nature, such as for example, "So-and-so hasn't seen a doctor for six months in this facility, why is that?" Or, "The doctor who saw so-and-so spent ten minutes with her and didn't check for bedsores, what can we do about that?" I do not mean to insult the reader's intelligence by giving such basic advice, but if advocates rush in without good information, their efforts may be doomed from the start.

Give people the opportunity to do what is right.
An advocacy principle that can provide balance and help avoid unnecessary conflict is that when possible, the people one is advocating against should be given the chance to do the right thing. That is, an advocate should not immediately assume that human service workers would not be fair and responsive. While it may be that the service system will not respond or provide what is needed, sometimes failure to respond is more a function of regulations or oppressive social policy than it is the actions of individual service workers. Also, unresponsiveness is often due to naiveté, incompetence, pride, and/or unconscious devaluation by individual human service workers. However, people cannot respond positively unless they have an idea of what a positive response might be. A citizen advocate should make her expectations clearly known, unless there is some good reason not to, and give people the opportunity to respond to those expectations. The advocate can always increase the vigor of her advocacy if needed, but sometimes people actually will do what they are asked to do.

Expect cooperation, but do not be surprised by resistance.
When an advocate speaks up for the interests of a particular protégé, the advocate may find that he or she is up against formidable forces in the protégé's life. When an advocate speaks up vigorously, the resistance from service providers may be equally vigorous. In fact, sometimes the response to advocacy may be disproportionately aggressive; for example, in response to simple questions or concerns, an advocate may be forbidden access to her protégé.

On occasion, one might encounter a service provider who appreciates the limits of the service system, and who therefore appreciates the watchfulness and advocacy of private citizens — but this is rare. More often, advocates will be met with defensiveness and resistance. Like most of us, administrators, bureaucrats, and service workers generally do not like being challenged or having demands made of them. Resistance can take a variety of forms. It may be passive, where one is told, "Thank you for bringing this to our attention; we'll get right on it," and then little or nothing happens. More active resistance may range from excuse-making to outright counter-attacks, such as accusing the advocate of having ignoble motives, or disparaging the advocate's reputation. Most people do not like change, especially when change means inconvenience. People may also resist out of pride. In the face of such resistance, advocates need to be prepared to hold their ground, and to escalate their advocacy efforts with careful, measured responses.

Advocates must bear in mind, however, that sometimes human service workers would like to respond, but are unable to do so because of limitations of the service system, lack of funding, or policies handed down from above. There may be understandable reasons why a service provider does not or cannot meet certain expectations, but that does not objectively change the reality of the situation for the protégé. A citizen advocate's role is to concentrate on "what," not "why." That is, the advocate must focus on what the person's actual situation is, rather than on the reasons that a human service provider may give for why something is like it is — even when those reasons are legitimate. Being clear about what a person's life is like in the present circumstances can sometimes lead to a new direction in resolving a problem. For example, some citizen advocates have given up on the human service system and instead brought the protégé to their own home. Or, advocates may push to higher levels of authority to create a solution that no one at lower levels could have thought possible.

Going against the stream in dealing with a powerful bureaucracy can be unpleasant. Advocates are often described by professional human service agencies as irrational, "too emotional," or "too attached." People in power do not like to be embarrassed or have their reputation put in jeopardy — who does? Also, as I have mentioned, there is always a danger that a service provider will retaliate against the protégé, whether consciously or unconsciously.

The nitty-gritty of advocacy is often eye-opening for advocates. We need not anticipate all that a citizen advocate might face, but suffice it to say that the independence of the advocate is a crucial element in raising a strong voice in the face of injustice. An advocate must be prepared to absorb some of the same devaluing responses that her protégé has had to contend with for years or even a lifetime.

A word of caution: advocacy for the sake of advocacy, or advocacy for the sake of working out some agenda on the advocate's part (revenge, anger, pride) is usually not helpful to the protégé. There is nothing about being an advocate that makes the citizen advocate morally superior or even necessarily right. The moral goodness or rightness of an advocate's actions must be objectively based on the best interests of the vulnerable person whose concerns and well-being are at stake. Advocates who pound on tables and raise their voices in self-righteous anger or pride can cause irreparable harm. An advocate may have a valid reason to pound on a table or raise his voice when more diplomatic efforts have failed, but generally an advocate will be far more effective with a careful, serious, respectful yet firm approach that gives people the chance to respond positively before stepping up to more adversarial advocacy methods.

Speak truth to power.
Sometimes citizen advocates have to confront powerful forces. It is therefore important that advocates speak from higher ground. That is, an advocate needs to base her advocacy on high-order principles that will withstand the defensiveness and counterarguments of service providers. For example, if an advocate is arguing for decent housing on behalf of an individual, landlords might argue that they do not have the resources for better housing conditions. Rather than argue over the question of resources, an advocate is on higher ground by maintaining a person's right to safe, decent housing at a fair cost. On another front, health care personnel may argue that a person's "quality of life" may be so poor that basic medical treatment should be denied. A higher ground would be to argue that the inherent value of a person's life is absolute rather than getting into arguments about the "quali-

ty" of a person's life.

These examples illustrate the importance of discerning the truth of a situation and speaking that truth when one is up against powerful forces. Sometimes those forces come tumbling down in the face of truth and turn out to be "paper tigers" — forces that only appeared to be powerful. This does not mean that truth will always prevail; an advocate will not always win. In the face of powerful forces, advocacy is more about witness than it is about winning. That is, an advocate may be the only person on the scene who sees something for what it is and speaks the truth. Whether or not people hear the truth — and whether or not they respond to it — is beyond the advocate's control.

Use enough advocacy, but not too much advocacy.
An advocate needs to gauge the amount of pressure necessary to accomplish what is needed. A simple analogy is, "never use a cannon when a pea-shooter will do." For example, making a request of a direct service worker or line supervisor is less antagonistic than going to the executive director, threatening lawsuits, or going to the press. Sometimes more vigorous advocacy is necessary to make things happen, but high-powered advocacy can have unwanted ramifications and can unnecessarily hurt naive or innocent people. Paradoxically, high-powered advocacy can hinder the citizen advocate's efforts unless more reasonable efforts have first been tried.

To gauge "how much" advocacy is needed, it can be helpful for an advocate, after some time has passed, to reflect on how the protégé has benefited (or not benefited) from her involvement in the protégé's life. Self-examination can sometimes lead one to become engaged in a deeper way, or a more practical way, or to identify other issues that need to be resolved before taking a specific advocacy action.

Persevere through trials and difficulties
Asking people to persevere is a little like telling them to go to the dentist. Advocates who persevere through difficult times, however, typically do so because they could not do anything else but remain steadfast. Abandoning someone they care about is simply not an

alternative they would consider. Perseverance is not a matter of "oh, you have so much patience," or "what a wonderful person you must be." Those kinds of responses are based on stereotypical views of people who must be so difficult to be with that one would have to be a saint to "put up" with them. Some people are difficult to be with, but in the vast majority of Citizen Advocacy relationships, people enjoy each other's company, they look forward to spending time together, and they miss one another when apart for a long time (e.g., Linda and Charlene). Even relationships that have times of great difficulty may also have times of great joy (e.g., Louisa and Teresa). Sometimes a relationship may be very difficult at the outset, but vastly improves over time (e.g., Diane and Aretha).

When the person being advocated for does make it difficult to stay in the relationship, citizen advocates should look beyond the present situation or circumstances and consider what lies behind the difficulty. For example, when Aretha was being rejecting, Diane did not walk away, but assumed that Aretha had reasons for her rejection. Perseverance involves moving forward even when — or especially when — one cannot be certain of what the outcome will be, and when there are reasons to believe one might fail, but one presses on regardless.

In some situations, citizen advocates who become engaged in a person's life reach a point where they have to ask themselves, "If I do not remain in this person's life, who will?" Perseverance in a Citizen Advocacy relationship is usually not about persevering with a protégé's faults and failings — although that may be part of it. The greater perseverance is needed in the face of the difficulties imposed by the social devaluation the person has endured.

When a citizen advocate is facing obstacles that seem insurmountable, it is helpful to keep the long-term perspective. Sometimes what is impossible in the present moment becomes possible later. Or, it may be that the benefits to a Citizen Advocacy relationship are completely different from what one first expected. Often the benefits of one's engagement may only come after a long period of time, perhaps many years.

Seek out support

A citizen advocate would do well to occasionally spend time, alone or with others, reflecting on who the person is for whom he or she is an advocate. Advocates find themselves facing situations they never would have imagined. For these and other reasons, advocates need support. This does not mean that advocates need to become quasi-professionals and advocacy experts. They need moral support, common sense and information.

Being a part of someone's life, and having influence in that person's life, are serious matters. This is especially true when one's actions, or one's failure to act, have consequences in a person's life. A key role of the Citizen Advocacy office is to assist citizen advocates to think through what their role and actions will be in what are sometimes very difficult situations.

A citizen advocate has, or should have, access to a Citizen Advocacy office that can provide such support, although the Citizen Advocacy office need not be the primary or even the most important source of support. Support from an advocate's own personal networks, such as family, friends and co-workers, has many advantages in that it builds upon natural ties and relationships, is likely to be available in the future, and it widens the circle of people involved in the protégé's life.

Seeking out support is particularly important when health issues are at stake. The dynamics and dangers that devalued people face in hospital settings or nursing homes will often present themselves in confusing, even deceptive ways, and having someone to talk to who understands those dynamics is extremely important.

Consider the lessons of personal engagement in the life of a devalued person as a learning journey and opportunity for personal growth

Opening one's life to a devalued person will bring unexpected lessons. One will not learn these lessons from books — including this one. Yet a person must be open in order to learn. Pride is a great obstacle to learning, and so true learning requires humility. For example, to stand before a person who has a mental handicap, a person who cannot read or write, has never read a book, has little knowledge of the ways of the world, and to regard that person as one's teacher takes humility. To set aside preconceived notions about what makes a person valuable calls one to be humble in the truest sense of the word.

CHAPTER FOURTEEN

The Look of Hope:
The Story of Sisa and Harold

One of the most difficult challenges we face in Citizen Advocacy is when someone with a disability, or their mother or father, looks at you with hope in their eyes. I am humbled by this look, for I fear I too will let them down. To step into their lives and offer new hope can be frightening — even dreadful. Whenever I meet a person who needs an advocate, I dread that I might become yet another faceless bureaucrat, another agency caseworker with a waiting list, another person making promises I might fail to keep. There are people for whom we could not find advocates, and even when we found one, sometimes our hopes, and theirs, were unrealized.

Yet sometimes Citizen Advocacy relationships fulfill our hopes beyond what we ever imagined, and we are surprised by the joy of two people becoming integral to one another's lives. Following is Sisa and Harold's story as told by Sisa Beckwith.

I am a wife and mother with three children of my own, a step-daughter, and I am expecting my fourth child. I'm originally from Maryland, and my husband's from New York. His work brought us to the Pittsburgh area, and we have lived here for seven years. We're active in the pro-life movement; in fact, I learned about Harold at a pro-life meeting. Adam Hildebrand, the Citizen Advocacy coordinator, came to the meeting and presented Harold's story. I didn't know he was going to be there. It was one of my first meetings that I attended with my husband, because he was staying out very late at those meetings. I thought I'd better start going with him. That way we can have more time together. So we had this meeting and Adam was giving this presentation. It seemed like he was talking to me more than to the others in the room, which made me a little uncomfortable, because we had never met before.

I'm going to get emotional, because hearing Harold's story just really touched my heart in such a profound way. I didn't expect it to affect me. Here is this man in his sixties in the nursing home, whose only family contact was his father up until four years ago, when his father passed away. We didn't even know if Harold knew that his father had died. Harold had no other family contact. Adam and Denise had asked people from Harold's former life to get involved. They said, "The Harold I knew died many years ago."

When I heard this, it bothered me that there was somebody — and now I know he's not the only one — who doesn't have anybody. He was just up there [in the nursing home] by himself. His only contact with another human being was a nurse. How friendly could that contact be?

So we walked out of the meeting and Richard, my husband, said, "So you are going to call them tomorrow, aren't you?" We had not talked about it. I said, "What are you talking about?" Richard answered, "You're going to call and become Harold's advocate." I got a little irritated. "What are you talking about? I don't have time for that. You know that's a life-long commitment they're asking." He says, "You have time. You can do it. I know you, you're going to call them." I said, "No, I'm not. I'm too busy. I got too many other things to do."

I did a Bible study that night and every Scripture I came across, which had nothing to do with Harold or anything, was telling me, "You're going to do this. This is what you are going to do." I'm thinking, "I've never been spoken to by the Lord like that." The

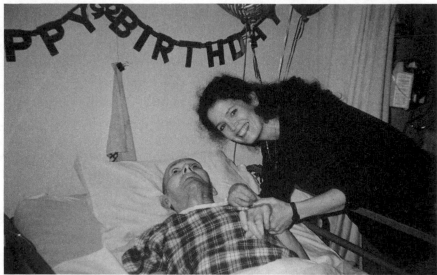

Harold and Sisa

next day, all morning I procrastinated. "I'm not going to call," I thought. "I'm just going to keep cleaning my house. I'll find other things to do." Finally I called. I just broke down and cried and said, "When can I meet Harold?"

That was on a Tuesday when I called, and Thursday evening I met Harold. It was November 1996. We've been going up to the nursing home — I haven't counted the times we've visited Harold, but we go as a family once a week. I go with one of my kids or by myself during the week. He's part of our family. When we say prayers at night, the children pray for Harold as part of our family. When people ask, "How many people are in your family?" Harold is among the people in our family.

Harold has severe multiple sclerosis, and he can't talk. After being with him for some time, I can communicate with him through his eyes, and sometimes he squeezes my hand, but it isn't a consistent response. I'm not really sure if it's a muscle reflex or what — he nods and shakes his head a lot — he can't control it. My kids asked me, "Why does Harold keep saying 'no'?" I said, "He's not saying no, that's just what his muscles do." We brought another member of our family to meet Harold, and my youngest daughter Ruby, who was four at the time, explained, "He's not saying 'no' to you, he just does that."

When I go by myself, I talk to him. I tell him what I've done the past couple days, and I usually hold his hand. If he has mail, like a statement from the nursing home, I open it and read it to him. I read books to him. Usually I have conversations with his room-mate, because his roommate can talk and likes to interrupt a lot. I try to be courteous, but I also try to let him know when he's cross-ing the line, because I'm there to visit Harold. I expect his room-mate to respect that.

Harold is bedridden, and I've asked the nurses if I could take him outside or if he could go to a church service. Their answer: "He's on bed rest." I asked, "Couldn't we put him on a gurney?" They looked at me like I had ten heads. So I think, "O.K., we'll just do what we can to bring life into his room." So that's what we do. When the kids come, they usually color. My oldest stepdaughter likes to read to him too. My other children color and they show him the pictures and he responds. His eyes get bigger. You can tell he's looking at the picture. If he was moving all the time, he stops moving to look at the picture. When my son Thomas would say something, like, "Hi," or Bye," Harold would turn his head. He knew Thomas was there. Thomas would sit on my lap, so I brought a stool to have something to sit on next to his bed. Thomas would play "take away" with Harold; he'd put something in Harold's hand, and then take it away. So there was interaction, physical interaction. My husband would come and sit and talk with Harold too. Our visits had a fam-ily atmosphere. Sometimes the kids would get a little rambunc-tious. I wondered if Harold were able to speak, he might say, "Get these kids out of my room!" Thomas found the button that makes the bed go up and down — I'm sure Harold doesn't like the sudden movement.

The nurses have commented a number of times that they have noticed a change in Harold. They said he seems more aware of peo-ple, that maybe he's looking for us, whether it's us or one of the nurses. The nurses seem to be interacting more with Harold, espe-cially this one nurse who was new. At first she came in and didn't say a word to Harold. She asked me if I was his daughter. I said, "no." She said, "Well, you look like the person in the picture there on the wall." I said, "Well, that is me, but I'm not his daughter." She didn't ask Harold how he was feeling today or anything. When she went to the other bed, she conversed with Harold's roommate. That made me angry. I was too angry to say anything. But now, that nurse has changed. She will say to Harold, "How you doing?" They call him "Doc." She'll say, "How you doing, Doc? You have a visitor today? Isn't that nice? Aren't the kids fun? They're so cute." They are treating him like a person now. They treat him like he's there, instead of somebody just coming in and changing a feeding tube or whatever. Harold is more responsive. He seems more aware that someone is there with him. I think he appreciates knowing someone is there. Sometimes I'll stand outside the room if he's facing the other way and watch him for a couple of minutes. He might be agitated, or what I'd call agitated, because his arms would be going and stuff like that. Then I'll go into the room, and he seems to calm down. He'll calm down and hold my hand. Usually his hand is in a fist, and now he opens his hands for me. He lets me clip his nails — when you hold your hand in a fist the fingernails dig in. So he lets me do that. I've made him a few flannel gowns, which gives him a little ownership.

When our family visits Harold, a lot of the other residents notice us because they see this family making an entrance, going down the hall, and everyone on the floor says "hello." We'll stop and talk to people, especially the people we know who rarely have family visits. There's one lady in the front of the hall with whom Amy has become friends — they play cards together. We have to set aside at least two hours when the whole family goes.

We celebrate Harold's birthday, and he knows when it's the kids' birthdays. They receive gifts from him, and we let him know that he gave them a gift. At Christmas, we have gifts from him that they open up there. Then we give him gifts. It's all part of the day.

When we first started getting to know Harold, my husband said that he sees Harold coming to our home; we'd like to take him out to our home for a holiday. Now I'm not sure. A lot would have to change for that to happen. I'm afraid that it would be such a big shock to his system. We'd like to take him out to the grassy area outside the nursing home. There's a nice gazebo-type area there.

But I think it would have to be a gradual thing, maybe just a little time outside near the door at first. It would take some time. It would be a miracle to have such a wonderful thing happen, to have him sitting on our deck.

I also heard of a new computer thing that's called "writing with your eyes." There's a laser that follows the pupil towards the letters that you're looking at, and it spells out everything. So I'm looking into getting more information about that.

When Harold's story was presented, Adam said something like, "Not only would you be a blessing in his life, but the blessings that come to you will be tenfold." That bothered me in the beginning. I thought, "I'm not in it for the blessings for me." I felt really strongly about that. After awhile, after a couple of months of seeing Harold on a regular basis, my husband and I were asking each other, "Do you sense something different?" Things were going almost too smoothly for us, with the whole family. The family atmosphere was a lot calmer and more peaceful. It was just a more peaceful time with the kids. That was one of the blessings. I thought, "Well, if that's the only blessing we get, it's a good one."

Everything seemed to be flowing a lot better — and to think I was concerned about the time I'd spend with Harold. A friend of mine had told me not to worry about the time. She said, "Think about him that day and the time would be there for you to go see him that day." That's how it's always worked. Being with Harold has affected us in so many ways. Other family members from out of town have gone up with us to see Harold.

Being Harold's advocate has taught me that a nursing home is not a place I want my parents to be. I've always told my mother that she would never be in a nursing home. No matter what we had to do, she would be in our home.

I can make a difference in one person's life. Other people at the nursing home light up when they see our family coming in. Even if it's just a simple "hello." It is amazing how a "hello" and a smile can change a person's whole day. When I receive a smile and a "hello," I really appreciate it. A nurse said to me one time, "You're always so happy when you come here. But if you had to be here every day ..." I said, "I hope that wouldn't change." But I understand that it does for the people who work there.

Author's Comments

What Sisa did for Harold was simply what families and loved ones do for one another. She shared herself and her family with Harold. Every Sunday after church, and often during the week, Sisa, her husband Richard, and their children went to the nursing home to see Harold, filling his room with life and love and laughter. Sisa established trust with the nursing staff, and asked questions. The cookies she sometimes brought to the nursing station and her friendly demeanor helped the nursing staff listen — and respond — to her questions. After Sisa had been spending time with Harold for a year or so, the nurses remarked to her, "You know, Harold is more alert these days, he's really perked up!" Harold had become more of a person in the eyes of the nursing home staff.

While spending time with Harold, Sisa learned subtle cues about what Harold felt. For example, most of the time Harold's hands were curled up in a fist. After visiting for some time, Sisa called us very excited, and said, "Harold opened his hand!" Harold's opening his hand was his way of saying to Sisa, "Yes, I want you in my life."

Sisa treated Harold as a human being, a person. She believed he understood everything she said to him. She touched him and looked into his eyes. She loved him. Her family loved him. He became a member of her family. In 1997, Sisa wrote the following words about her relationship with Harold for our newsletter at One to One: Citizen Advocacy:

> Imagine . . . lying in a white bed with white sheets, looking at white walls, wearing faded hospital gowns, day after day, week after week, year after year . . . The man in the next bed has a TV, a radio, everyday clothes to wear, weekly if not daily visits from family and friends, and his walls

are covered to the ceiling with cards, photos, and art work. Harold doesn't have any of this because he is the man lying in the bed with white sheets, looking at white walls, and wearing faded hospital gowns for the past eight years. Harold has advanced multiple sclerosis and has very little use of his body. Harold's father was his only visitor until two years ago when his dad died. Harold had no one else in his life.

I heard about Harold through Citizen Advocacy when Adam Hildebrand spoke at a community meeting. I wanted to do something, but was afraid. My husband Richard encouraged me to pray about becoming an advocate for Harold. So I did. While praying for Harold and for guidance, a scripture passage came to mind and has since been written on my heart: "I tell you the truth, whatever you did for one of the least of these brothers of mine, you did for me." Matt. 25:40

Never had a scripture spoken so loud and clear. The next morning I made a phone call to One to One: Citizen Advocacy, and met with Adam Hildebrand and his associate, Denise Shaw. We met and discussed Harold, and later in the week, went to meet him.

Today, the Geriatric Center where Harold lives has become an extension of our home. My husband, Richard, and our four children Jacqueline (9), Amy (6), Ruby (4), and Thomas (18 months) have embraced Harold as part of our family. Initially, I visited with Harold by myself, but now he sees the whole family every Sunday after church, and I visit with him during the week. Time spent with Harold is filled with love, laughter, and the children's constant chatter. On quieter visits I read to Harold and hold his hand, which isn't easy because it is usually in a fist or shaking, but after some gentle coaxing, he opens his hand for me.

My daughters didn't like the fact that Harold didn't have anything on his walls. So the little artists went to work. Harold now views artwork, which includes flowers with hearts, "I love you messages," and a picture Amy drew of

Harold in his bed with everyone around him. Although Harold's bed still has white sheets, it now has a colorful blanket on it.

We celebrated Harold's 63rd birthday, with cake and ice cream. I made him a couple of plaid flannel hospital gowns, which he seems to like. The nurses who care for Harold have shared with me that they have noticed a change in him — although he cannot speak — he seems to be more aware and notices when someone comes into the room. Every time a nurse tells me that Harold seems different since my coming to meet him, tears fill my eyes and I thank God for Harold ...

I have learned not to be afraid. I am now not afraid to help someone like Harold. My children are learning not to be afraid. They are learning how to open their heart to someone outside of their family who may be different. My husband and I hope that our children are learning that "you have to take care of your own."

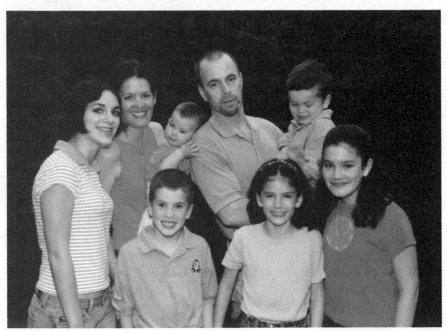

The Beckwith Family

The birthday party Sisa mentioned above had memorable moments. Sisa had invited Denise Shaw and me to share in the celebration. We do not know when Harold last had a real birthday party. Julie Clarke, a friend and a Citizen Advocacy coordinator from Wollongong, Australia, was visiting One to One at the time, so we invited her along.

Sisa had brought the birthday cake to the nursing home earlier in the day and asked the nurses to hold the cake at the nurse's station until it was time for the party. Written on the top of the box were the words, "Save for Harold's family." Julie pointed the box out to me, with a big smile and tears in her eyes. Sisa and her family were Harold's family. They knew it, the nurses knew it, we knew it, Harold knew it — and families celebrate birthdays.

Sisa later became a board member at One to One, and from time to time we asked her to share her story. Whenever Sisa began to speak about Harold, tears welled up in her eyes. These were not tears of pity, or of pain, but tears of love and joy. The words that Sisa spoke were plain and simple: how her children loved Harold, how Harold became more relaxed when she was with him, how most of the nurses treated Harold better because she was in his life. These were simple, ordinary words, but words made extraordinary by the love with which they were spoken.

During one of our many conversations about Harold, Sisa remarked, "You know, Richard and I have noticed lately that we have more peace in our household now that we are spending time with Harold. We think that Harold has helped improve our marriage. He is giving us peace."

One morning a few years after Sisa met Harold, she called me and said, "Harold's leg is broken. Someone broke his leg." In shock and anger, she asked, "How could they do that? How could they be so careless?" I didn't have any answers, all I could do was listen and share her frustration. We talked about how to try to find out what happened. Sisa asked lots of questions, but got few answers. Harold's legs were pulled up close to his body from multiple sclerosis (MS), and his bones were brittle. Someone apparently moved him too quickly, or with too much force, probably while changing his bed. Whoever did it may not even have realized what happened. Maybe it was an honest mistake. Maybe the nurse's aide was in a hurry, or maybe it took very little force to break his leg, or maybe it was simple carelessness in shifting his body — we will never know what really happened. We hoped that asking questions had some effect. Maybe the aides would be more careful.

During the last months of his life, Harold was having difficulty digesting his food. Sisa spoke with a doctor-friend of hers about Harold's MS, and contacted the local MS society to ask how multiple sclerosis affects the digestive system. She learned that in the final stages of MS, it is common for the digestive system to stop functioning due to deterioration of the nervous system. The nursing home put Harold on total parenteral nutrition, which supplies nutrition directly into the blood stream through a tube. This helped, but Harold was becoming progressively weaker. A few months later, on January 6, 2001, Harold died at the age of 64, when his bodily systems failed.

Sisa arranged for a memorial service for Harold, and invited Denise, myself, and a couple of board members from One to One and other friends to come. Rev. Dr. Michael Hoover, the doctor-friend who gave Sisa advice and support from time to time, is also a deacon in the Roman Catholic Church, and agreed to conduct a memorial service.

We gathered at the non-denominational chapel at the nursing home, thinking that some of the nurses might attend, but they didn't come. Sisa's daughter Amy played Bach's Musette *on the violin. Deacon Hoover led us in prayer, and Sisa and I shared a couple of readings from Scripture. After the readings, those gathered shared their thoughts and feelings. There were tears, laughter, sorrow, and joy — Harold's final gifts to us as we gathered to honor his memory.*

A person's name can have great meaning. Deacon Hoover gave the homily, during which he reflected on Harold's name and nick-names: Harold, "Reed," and "Doc." A "herald" is one who announces great news, one who speaks with an important voice, and whose message, as we remember from the song "Hark, the herald angels sing," is one of great joy. From "Reed," Deacon Hoover recalled the scripture "a bruised reed He shall not break" (Isaiah 42:3). As Reed, Harold was crushed and alone for many years, but not broken. The inner core of Harold's being remained intact, his human spirit never lost. As "Doc," Harold was a learned person, a doctor of a kind of knowledge unknown to most people. His learning was not from books or from typical human experience, but from what he learned through his suffering.

By worldly standards, Harold had lost everything; everything, that is, but the capacity to give love and receive love — a gift beyond measure. I do not know if Harold was an intelligent man, or if he was a thoughtful man. I do know that he loved Sisa, and he loved Sisa's family. Harold brought a communion of love to Sisa and her family, and indirectly, to me. What greater lesson is there to learn? Harold taught us by the pure essence of his being.

I never heard Harold speak a word, never heard the sound of his voice, but I heard his message. His message, as Harold's life spoke to us, is living testimony that every life is precious, and sacred. Harold taught us many important lessons. By his mere presence, his very being, stripped of all the externals of life, Harold taught us that love is what makes us distinctively human. He taught us that it is in giving that we receive, and that love is deeper than words, or intelligence, or human acts. These mysteries, hidden from the wise, are revealed to us through wounded people.

CHAPTER FIFTEEN

The Story Behind Sisa and Harold's Story

Every Citizen Advocacy relationship has a "behind the scenes" story. Often it takes months–and occasionally, years — to find the right advocate. For Harold, it took us four years to find the right person. During those years, the look of hope in the eyes of Harold's father often kept me awake at night. After two unsuccessful attempts at matching Harold, I felt we had failed. Fortunately, what had been a source of deep personal anguish eventually became a story of transforming love and commitment.

Harold was 55 when we met him, and had lived in a large nursing home since he was about 40. Before I became involved in Citizen Advocacy, I had volunteered at this same nursing home by leading a Bible study group, so I knew the activities director. I was able to walk around freely and meet people, since most of the staff thought I was a minister from having seen me walk the halls with a Bible in my hand.

In 1989, as relatively inexperienced Citizen Advocacy coordinators, Denise Shaw and I went to the nursing home and asked the activities director if she could tell us about people with disabilities who might need an advocate. She gave us a list, and we went about the nursing home visiting the people named. We noticed, however, that everyone we were seeing already had people in their lives. Most had afghans on their beds and personal decorations around their room, signs that family members or others were involved. Most were fairly capable, able to walk, talk, and care for themselves. In fact, most were not even in their rooms, and were instead in the recreation areas or in the cafeteria. It dawned on us that the activities director had suggested people who in her mind were those an advocate would enjoy spending time with — people with mild impairments who could walk, talk and carry on a conversation.

We decided to pitch the list and look for people who had no personal decorations or cards on the wall or on the nightstand by their bed. When we saw how barren Harold's room was, we assumed no one was visiting him. Harold was unable to speak and had little or no control over his body. While I believe he understood what people said to him, he was unable to communicate what he understood.

A nurse's aide told us what little she knew of Harold's background, and that his elderly father occasionally visited him. We learned that Harold was Harold, Jr., and that he grew up in the same town I had. To my amazement, I realized that Harold's father and my father had worked together in the steel mill, and were both foremen in the same department. I remember my father talking about "Doc," a nickname for Harold's father, which Harold shared. We visited Harold several times at the nursing home to get a sense of who he was. Harold had a lot of involuntary movement, and often shook his head from side to side, as if he were saying "no." When I met Harold, I said to him, "Harold, I believe that you can understand me." When I said that, Harold looked into my eyes ever so briefly. I explained Citizen Advocacy to Harold, and told him that we would go see his father.

Initially Harold's father was confused by our interest in Harold. Since he knew my father, however, he was willing to talk. Though there is much we were never able to learn about Harold, his father told us some things about his son's life. He told us that Harold had been married, had children, divorced, and had been a truck driver. When he was 38 years old, Harold was driving a truck cross-country when his legs began to bother him. He pulled his truck over on the interstate and called his father because he couldn't drive home. After numerous tests, Harold was diagnosed with multiple sclerosis (MS), which progressed rapidly. Harold lived with his father and stepmother for a number of years, but after his stepmother died, he went to the nursing home.

Harold's father was 82 when we met, and was no longer able to drive to visit Harold. He visited his son when someone could take him, but that was not very often. Talking with Harold's father over coffee at his dining room table, he stopped during the conversation for a moment and asked, "What will happen to my son when I die? Who will care about what happens to him?" The question hung in the air for a moment. I took a deep breath and promised him we would try to find an advocate. I said, "I don't know if we will find someone who cares the way you do, but I assure you we will try." Harold's father gave me a look of hope.

We visited with Harold again. I told him that his father and my father worked together in the steel mill, and that his father was unable to visit as often as he would like. I told him more about Citizen Advocacy, and that we wanted to find someone who could spend time with him, someone who would care about what happened to him. I asked him if that was all right with him. I do not know what Harold thought about what I said, but I hoped he understood me. I said that while I could not be sure what he wanted, since his father wanted us to find an advocate, we would try to find one.

We talked with a former neighbor of Harold's to see if we could identify someone from his past who might become re-involved. The neighbor told us of an old friend of Harold's, and said Harold and this friend were at one time inseparable. I phoned him, but he was upset by my call and clearly wanted to be left alone. He said: "Harold is curled up like a baby and is not the person he used to be. I would not be able to deal with that. Harold died a long time ago."

When I heard those words, "Harold died," I sat at my desk, stunned. I grieved the loss of a friendship that could have meant so much — but was now lost. Harold was not dead, but the friendship was. I wanted to tell Harold's friend that Harold is alive, that he is still in this world, and that he still needs him. I wanted to tell him that true friendship should endure change. I wanted to let him know that Harold was still Harold. Ultimately, I had to let go of my feelings and avoid judging Harold's friend.

A few months after we met Harold, we matched him with a woman who visited him for about a year. This relationship consisted of occasional visits, but we never sensed much of a connection between this advocate and Harold. She later moved out of the area.

About a year later, we again tried matching Harold, this time with a man. We felt this match had potential. Soon after we matched them, however, the advocate began having health problems. For a while, doctors suspected that *he* might have MS. This made it impossible for him to spend time with Harold, whose MS was quite advanced.

After two failed matches, we were at a standstill. This lasted over a year. While Harold remained on our working list — which is a list of five or six people for whom we are recruiting advocates at a given time — we were at a loss. Feeling we had failed made us afraid of failing again. During this time, we were also learning more about the increasing threats to the lives of highly vulnerable people in nursing homes. Harold was on a feeding tube. Might a decision be made at some point to "withdraw life support"?

When I visited other Citizen Advocacy programs, gave talks to community groups, or met with people interested in Citizen Advocacy, I talked about how we believed in the value of every person's life. I said that every person was important, no matter how vulnerable or impaired. When I'd say those things, I'd think of Harold and feel like a hypocrite. The longer it took to find the right person for Harold, the worse I felt.

I had promised Harold — and Harold's father — that we would do our best to find someone. The personal connection between my father and Harold's father made me feel an even greater obligation. I felt if I could not find an advocate for Harold, maybe I shouldn't do this work any more. Maybe I no longer had what it takes to be a Citizen Advocacy coordinator. Maybe it was time for me to step aside. Maybe the board should find someone who really believed there was someone out there for Harold.

Then I got to the heart of the problem. I asked myself if *I* really believed that Harold's life was just as important as anyone else's life. It wasn't just nursing home personnel who may not recognize

Harold's dignity as a human being. Maybe *I* didn't mean it when I said that every person's life is sacred. Did I really believe that Harold's life had value? Did I believe that someone would care about what happens to Harold? Was I guilty of thinking of Harold as not as important as other people for whom we were recruiting advocates? Was there a hidden place inside me that did not value Harold? That question frightened me the most. If that was true, if Harold's life was not equally as important as any other person's life, including my own, I really was a hypocrite.

I believe what I say about the dignity of every person's life, but do I always incorporate that belief into everything I say and do? No. As imperfect human beings, we all fall short of having absolute respect for *every* human being. For Harold, I had to rise above my imperfections and challenge my own hidden and ever-so-subtle devaluing tendencies. I had to search my heart and soul and ask myself if I truly believed in Harold's inherent dignity. If I was going to convince a potential advocate of Harold's absolute value as a human being, I first had to believe my own words.

Regarding the first two failed matches for Harold, I can think of a long list of "should-haves." I should have known better. I should have been more thorough. I should have asked more questions. I should have been clearer about what we were looking for in an advocate. I should have discussed what we were asking an advocate to do in greater depth.

Recognizing mistakes and taking responsibility for them is important. Mistakes have consequences. We might have known after a few conversations with the first advocate that, at the time, she did not have enough stability in her life to be there for Harold over the long haul. In our rush to find an advocate for Harold, we overlooked the obvious. Hindsight is wonderful, but good matching requires foresight. Human beings are complex, and relationships between human beings fragile. In the second match we made for Harold, there were not as many "should-haves." We could not have known that this advocate might possibly have MS.

There were two things that kept me from not giving up on Harold. First, there was Harold himself. I had looked into Harold's eyes and promised him we would try to find an advocate. Secondly,

I had promised Harold's father. I promised to try to find someone who would be there when he was gone. I can't say which haunted me more, the ever-so-brief look in Harold's eyes, or the look of hope in the eyes of his father. Both looks convicted me.

When we find ourselves at a standstill, it is helpful to re-examine our understanding of who is the person for whom we are recruiting an advocate and ask ourselves new questions. Considering Harold's extreme vulnerability, Denise and I discussed Harold's need for someone who would defend his life. To our knowledge, this particular nursing home was not withdrawing feeding tubes from people merely because they were severely impaired, but we were hearing accounts of such things happening elsewhere. We needed to find someone who had a high regard for the intrinsic value of each human life, someone who believed that *every* life is sacred. We discussed how an advocate for Harold needed to be serious-minded and not afraid of serious challenges. We made a list of people and groups to approach, and on the list was the local pro-life organization. I knew a couple of people involved in this group, so I called and asked if I could make a fifteen-minute presentation at their next meeting.

As I reflected on what to tell them, I thought about how Harold was living in a world where the value of his life was not fully recognized. I recalled how a nurse's aide came into his room one time while I was visiting, and moved Harold into a different position without saying a word to him or acknowledging him in any way. Harold was being treated as if he were no longer "there." It is not unusual for people with advanced neurological impairments to be described as being "out of it." If Harold was no longer Harold, as his former friend believed, then Harold was only his body. These thoughts may not have been conscious on the part of the aide, or anyone else at the nursing home. Her actions, however, told me that she did not see Harold as a person, but as a body without personality or spirit. The reality for Harold was that he was no longer seen as fully human.

With these thoughts in the forefront of my mind, I went to the pro-life meeting. I was not thinking of my presentation as advocate recruitment per se, but as a way of finding people who could lead us to someone who might become Harold's advocate. Advocate recruitment usually happens through one-to-one, face-to-face discussions. These were serious people in front of me, and I hoped they would lead us to someone who would sit down with us and talk more in-depth about Harold's life.

I told the people at the meeting that there was a purpose for Harold's life. I told them I was looking for someone who believed that every life is sacred, and who was willing to act on that belief. I remember saying, "Right up the road from here, only a mile away, lies a man whose life is sacred, but most people regard him, consciously or unconsciously, as less than human." Here was an opportunity to live out one's belief in the sanctity of human life. The value of his life did not depend on his ability to speak, to engage in a relationship, or even to think. His life had value not in what he did, but in who he was — a human being.

I described the role of an advocate as affirming Harold's identity as a human being. Harold was a forgotten person, and to some people, no longer a person. When a person is no longer thought of as human, inhumane things happen. I was looking for someone who would worry about this for Harold, someone who would ask questions about his care, someone who would love Harold.

I also described how an advocate would benefit from knowing Harold, even though I found this hard to define. I took a leap of faith and said: "Harold's life has a purpose; you will be blessed by knowing him."

I noticed that one person at the meeting, Sisa, was particularly engaged in what I was saying. She took in every word, and did not avert her eyes as people often do when I am talking with a small group. I remember wishing I could take her aside and talk to her about Harold.

Sisa called me the next morning and said, "I have to meet Harold." We made arrangements to meet with Sisa to talk about Harold, and about Citizen Advocacy. When we orient a new advocate, we usually spend a fair amount of time talking through a number of issues and topics: who the person is, what is going on in his life, the patterns of the common life experiences of devalued people, the principles of Citizen Advocacy, the nature and role of advocacy, and how the advocate might begin to form a relationship. This information is shared through informal, one-to-one discussions, and the advocate may hardly realize that he or she is being "oriented" in a formal sense. Our purpose is to help the advocate get off to a good start in the relationship, to help the advocate gain a basic understanding of Citizen Advocacy, and to develop a relationship with the advocate ourselves.

We met with Sisa and told her what we knew of Harold's background, and about what kind of role she might assume as an advocate. We also talked at some length about Citizen Advocacy. I confess that we moved through orientation with Sisa a little too quickly — we were anxious for Sisa to meet Harold. In the months and years to come, however, we had many discussions with Sisa by sharing the journey of her relationship with Harold.

Introducing Sisa to Harold was a turning point in my career as a Citizen Advocacy coordinator. The person who was among the most forgotten, and the most vulnerable, turned out to be one of the most important matches we ever made. I was renewed. I remember thinking, "Yes, I can do this. It is an honor and a privilege to do this work." We kept our promise to a lonely man worried about his son. Most important, we kept the promise we made to Harold. In Citizen Advocacy, we usually write what we call a "match letter" to new advocates. Following is the text of the letter we wrote to Sisa:

November 12, 1996
Dear Sisa,

We want you to know how encouraged we are that you are becoming an advocate for Harold. Your heartfelt, enthusiastic response is an answer to prayer — we have been looking for you for quite some time. You have already embarked on a learning experience with Harold, and we look forward to learning with you as your relationship develops.

Harold is one of the most vulnerable people whom we have matched with an advocate, given his degree of disability, and given the abandonment and isolation he has experienced. Indeed, in the minds of at least some people,

Harold is not even regarded as a person anymore, a person who experiences feelings, emotions, desires, needs.

Perhaps your most fundamental role in Harold's life is in a real sense to give him back his personhood. You have already begun to do just that by holding positive beliefs and assumptions about who he is. At the most fundamental level, Harold is a living, breathing, child of God. His life has meaning and purpose. Whether or not he ever communicates with you, whether or not you get anything back from him, we believe there is a purpose in Harold's life.

We cannot know all of what that purpose is, but part of it is what he will bring to you and your family. In sharing your love and your family with Harold, there will be many unexpected blessings. In helping Harold to regain his personhood, you are in essence upholding the basic principle that we are *all* God's children, and that the world's definition of what it means to be human falls short of the identity and sanctity of *every* human life.

As we've discussed, we will be on this journey with you, and we hope that you will feel free to call upon us at any time for encouragement, advice (knowing that you don't have to take it!) and support.

CHAPTER SIXTEEN

Values and Virtues That Can Help Sustain
Personal Engagement

Anyone who becomes involved in Citizen Advocacy will need to hold
certain basic values: that responding to someone in need is a good
thing, that human beings bear some responsibility towards one
another, that personal commitment has value, and that all people
should be treated with respect and afforded justice. Beyond these
basic values, people who become engaged in Citizen Advocacy —
especially those who do so over a long period of time — may discern
realities about human nature and about the world that challenge
them to take a deeper look at who they are and what they believe.

The purpose of this chapter is to explore concepts that I have
found to strengthen personal commitments between valued and
devalued people. I offer these concepts in the spirit of exploring
insights that I believe are true, but I do not presume that one must
believe as I do to be involved or effective in Citizen Advocacy. As
you read the following chapters, you may find that you do not share
some of the values or assumptions I will describe. I would encourage you to take in what you find helpful, and allow the rest to pass
by — or perhaps take another look at what I say at a later time.
Values and virtues must be embraced, not imposed, and so I invite
you to consider the ideas in this chapter as food for thought, and
then make up your own mind about what you believe.

In an ideal world, all the help that people with disabilities need would be naturally forthcoming and freely available from personal supporters and allies. In a perfect world, relationship-making enterprises like Citizen Advocacy would not be necessary. But we do not live in that world. In the world that we live in, we need to reclaim our ability to respond to basic human needs without making those needs an exclusive professional commodity of the human service industry.

The 30+ year history of Citizen Advocacy has proven that individual citizens will respond to the needs and interests of devalued people. When people become voluntarily engaged in the lives of individual devalued people through clear, conscious commitments, their engagement is more likely to last, and more likely to bear fruit. Without a conscious commitment, when forces emerge that make personal engagement difficult, relationships may fall apart or never take hold in the first place.

Most human relationships begin without a lot of clear thinking behind them. Usually people are drawn together by common interests and circumstances, and only later discover the meaning and purpose for being in and continuing a relationship. However some forms of communal relationships, such as intentional communities and faith communities, have very clear rationales and values that bind them together. On a more informal level, people who form deep alliances share values that build lasting bonds. I have observed a number of distinct but interrelated value perspectives that motivate people to become engaged in Citizen Advocacy:

- A perspective that places high value on human relationships, with an emphasis on belonging, love, and personal connection.

- A personal justice perspective, in which an advocate feels a sense of personal outrage and concern over how a particular devalued individual has been wrongly treated.

- A social responsibility perspective, in which people feel a responsibility to give something back to their community, especially to vulnerable or needy members of that community.

- A spiritual perspective, and in our western culture, usually (but not exclusively) a Judeo-Christian world-view. This perspective emphasizes an active love of one's neighbor as an expression of knowing, loving, and serving God.

- A social justice perspective, with a focus on human equality, fairness, and "giving to each his due." This perspective focuses on enabling people to attain and have what is good, right and fair.

- A community-building perspective, with an emphasis on making our communities safer, better places to live so that vulnerable people will have better, safer lives.

- A social change perspective, in which the emphasis is on changing social structures through the relationships that hold those structures together.

These perspectives are not exclusive of one another, and most people ascribe some value to several or even all of them, although usually there is an emphasis on one over and above the others. Many people may not be conscious at first of the values that motivate them to become personally engaged in the life of someone with a disability. Quite often, people discover a growing awareness of their motivations through personal action and reflecting on the values that support those actions.

Four Pillars that Support Personal Engagement in the Lives of Socially Devalued People

The values that people hold can strengthen or weaken personal engagements. I have said that engagement in Citizen Advocacy raises questions like "Who am I?" and, "What do I believe?" The remainder of this chapter deals, at least in part, with my response to those and similar questions. I share these insights not so much as an attempt to convert people to my way of understanding the world, but rather to propose (but not impose) values and virtues that can strengthen personal engagement between valued and devalued people, such as promoted by Citizen Advocacy. These might be thought of as "pillars," which can strengthen and uphold relationship commitments. The first two pillars are human values: 1) respect for the inherent dignity of every human being; and 2) the recognition that every human life is sacred. The second two pillars are human virtues: 1) love of neighbor; and 2) the promotion of justice.

I again emphasize that one need not accept or even understand these values and virtues to be involved in Citizen Advocacy: they are not foundational to the Citizen Advocacy concept. However, these ideas often do lead people to become, and remain, engaged in one another's lives, and to actions that defend and promote the well-being of vulnerable people.

Human Dignity

The decision to respond to another human being implicitly affirms that the other person has value. Most people rightly recoil at the thought of measuring the value of a human being. I believe that in truth, every human being is a unique, precious and irreplaceable individual whose life has intrinsic dignity.[23]

The word "dignity" is losing its meaning in our culture. We hear this word used in "death with dignity," or "dignity of choice," terms that imply that human dignity has something to do with unrestrained and unfettered freedoms that human beings want and expect in the course of their lives. However, this kind of dignity is license, not freedom. Misguided choices, divorced from any clear morality outside of the individual person, are an affront to the true dignity of human beings. This is selfish individualism, which defaces human dignity, as when people choose to pursue their own interests without regard for the interests of others or without regard for moral laws that safeguard and protect human dignity. We need to reclaim the true meaning of human dignity.

I believe that the dignity or worth of a human being is rooted in

---

[23] May, W. E. (1991). *An Introduction to Moral Theology.* Huntingdon, IN: Our Sunday Visitor Publishing Division, p. 23.

a mystery. When a human being comes into existence, a new, irreplaceable, unique and precious soul is created. Human procreation is itself a mystery. The creation of a new human soul is in essence the creation of something out of nothing. This soul has an indestructible quality, and once created, will exist for all eternity. I believe that the light of life that infuses that soul, and which unites it to a physical body so that the soul and body become a living unity, is a reflection of God who is the source of all light, truth, and goodness.

In this view, a person with a physical or mental impairment has the same intrinsic dignity and worth as every other human being. No matter how impaired or vulnerable a person may be, his life has inherent worth. An impairment of body or mind does not limit the capacity of the human spirit. It is in the human spirit, in a person's soul, where human dignity resides. Dr. Wolfensberger describes the nature of human dignity:

> The worth or dignity of a human being cannot be measured on any quantitative scale. That is, no one human being has any more, or less, value or worth than any other human being. The "worth" or dignity of a human lies in its mere existence, and is not something that one attains, earns, achieves, develops, or becomes. No one moment of human life is any more or less valuable than any other moment, from beginning to end. Human dignity does not depend on ability, intelligence, gender, bodily impairment, or any other characteristic. Human dignity is not measured by how much one suffers, or by how much one causes others to suffer. Just as human dignity cannot be attained or achieved, neither can it be lost or taken away. Human dignity, therefore, does not depend on one's ability to live autonomously, to make choices, or even to engage in human acts.[24]

---

[24] Adapted from a presentation by Wolf Wolfensberger at a workshop entitled: "The common life experiences of devalued (and especially handicapped) people, with a special emphasis on the growing threats to their lives," at a workshop in October, 1999, in Pittsburgh, Pennsylvania.

Today, the assaults against human dignity are many. The people most at risk are those deemed to have less social value and usefulness in our culture. Such people include handicapped babies (born or unborn), severely disabled people, elderly people, people who are chronically or terminally ill, and many other devalued groups.[25] When socially devalued people are no longer perceived as having essential, fundamental dignity and value, then justice to them is no longer required. When the essential value of a person's life no longer finds sanctuary in human dignity, then other standards of value — such as the "quality" of one's life — will fill the vacuum where human dignity once stood. We often see this played out in the lives of devalued people. Human dignity provides an impetus to defend, protect and preserve the life whose dignity is inviolable. We often see this in the actions of citizen advocates. Without this sense of inviolability, violence and injustice against vulnerable human beings expresses itself in many forms, and those whose dignity is denied, diminished, or devalued are the first among us to bear the consequences.

The Sacredness of Human Life

The essential dignity or worth of a human being is rooted in the sacredness of human life. A number of years ago, I invited Kim, a citizen advocate, and Michelle, her protégé, who was twelve years old, to accompany me to a conference in Seattle to help me give a talk on Citizen Advocacy. I had the good sense to give my talk before Michelle gave hers, because I knew that Michelle would be a hard act to follow. Michelle had good things to say about Citizen Advocacy, but the Citizen Advocacy talk was simply a platform from which Michelle gave a message that went to the very core of why we do what we do in Citizen Advocacy. Michelle has cerebral palsy, uses a wheelchair, and speaks in a soft, clear voice. During her talk, there was a moment when she stopped, looked out over

---

[25] See Wolfensberger, W. (1992). *The New Genocide of Handicapped and Afflicted People* (rev. ed.). Syracuse, NY: Author. See also Smith, W. (2000). *Culture of Death: The Assault on Medical Ethics in America.* San Francisco: Encounter Books.

the crowd of 200 or so people, and spoke these words ever so gently: "Life is precious." In that moment, a spirit fell over the room. Everyone present reflected on the preciousness of life, spoken by a child who knew something that many adults never discover — that life is precious, and indeed, sacred.

If we understand the word "sacred" as meaning, "set apart," then to say that human life is sacred means that human life is set apart from all other forms of life. In some respects, the pillar of human dignity and the pillar of the sanctity of human life are the same pillar. I make a distinction between human dignity and the sanctity of human life as separate but related pillars out of respect for people who may not ascribe to a sense of the sacred, and who therefore would not relate to the concept of the sanctity of human life. The sacredness of human life can be partially understood in secular terms (i.e., without reference to a spiritual worldview), but generally, to say that life is sacred means that it is set apart by its relationship to a divine entity. In Judeo-Christian terms, this is explained as mankind made in the image of God.

Whatever our perspective, to say that human life is sacred means that human life is precious and unique. If one believes this, then one is called to promote and defend the life of fellow human beings, and act with vigilance and determination when a person's life may be at stake. The sacredness of a person's life also has relevance for the ordinary, everyday moments of life. When our daily interactions are infused by a belief that the person before us — regardless of type or degree of impairment — is a human being whose life is sacred, those interactions become transformed by a virtuous regard for the sacredness of every human life.

Love of One's Neighbor

In our modern culture, love has become a flimsy, elastic word that means almost anything, or nothing. Yet in truth, love is the greatest human virtue.[26] Love is not just a feeling or emotion; it is an act of the will to desire the good of another. While not all Citizen

---

[26] See 1 Corinthians 13:13 ("Love is patient, love is kind . . . ") a Bible passage which non-Christians, agnostics, and even atheists can appreciate.

Advocacy alliances are based on human bonds of affection, this broader definition of love — seeking the good of the other person — can be said to always apply.

In Citizen Advocacy, citizens are invited into the lives of people who sometimes have no one who loves them. When a human connection is formed between an advocate and a devalued person, what might have been a story of utter abandonment may become instead a story of fidelity, courage, commitment and love. This is not a starry-eyed notion that assumes that love can heal all wounds, solve all problems, or eliminate suffering; it is a realization that love shares suffering. Love shares one another's burdens, and it is love that sustains people in the face of great difficulty.

Love that seeks the good of the other person for its own sake is a gift that one cannot earn, merit, or produce. Love is the giving of oneself to another without regard for what one might receive in return. If one is loving a person because that person makes one feel good, or because there is some advantage to oneself, that is a selfish love, which in the long run, will not last. After the good feelings pass, and after the selfish motives surface, people may discover that they have acted in ways more to please themselves than others.

Love, like other human virtues, becomes stronger with exercise. When we exercise our will to love, our capacity for love is strengthened. Love is the light of the soul that brings life to all other human virtues. Love enables us to hope, and hope enables us to hold on to faith — faith in the meaning of human existence, faith in the purpose of our lives, and faith in who we are and what we mean to one another. The source of this love, the light of faith, is Love in the highest sense, Love that many call God.

Justice

The concept of justice exudes a sense of integrity, fairness, and equality, and has deep historical roots. However, the dictionary definition of justice, "to give to each his due," is dry, legalistic and lifeless. Justice does mean a fair distribution of resources — giving each his due — but I am using justice here in a deeper sense to explain *why* we should give others their due. An adapted version of the classical definition of justice by Thomas Aquinas is: "the per-petual will to ensure that each person is given what is his due, what each person rightly deserves, by virtue of being human."[27] Promoting justice for someone who has been unjustly treated should be based on a conviction that every human being should be treated with respect and dignity, and that all people, regardless of disability or social condition, deserve what is right, good and fair.

Justice is the virtue of seeking the good of other people, which is love in action. The virtue of justice, grounded in love and compas-sion, results in outrage (rightful anger) when another person — especially one who is vulnerable — is treated wrongly and unfair-ly. A just person finds injustice against a vulnerable person intoler-able, and is compelled to right the wrong being done. As a human virtue, justice, like love, becomes stronger with practice. The above explanation of justice may help us understand what justice is, but it does not explain *why* one should promote justice. Why should we treat one another fairly? The dignity of each and every human being provides the fundamental reason for justice.

A citizen advocate can promote justice by upholding and uplift-ing a person's dignity in any and every way possible. For example, when we recruited Sisa for Harold, he did not have any regular clothes but only wore hospital gowns. Sisa saw to it that he had ordinary clothes to wear. She insisted on referring to Harold by his proper name rather than by a nickname adopted by the nursing home staff. She made sure that his personal hygiene was attended to, so that he would look and feel better about himself. These may seem like small things, but Sisa's respect for Harold's dignity helped others to treat him with respect. As a result, Harold got bet-ter medical care, which may have helped extend his life, and cer-tainly helped him live a better life.

Treating a person with dignity is a very real and substantial means to promoting justice. It creates an expectation, a demand that a person be given the respect that is due to every human being.

---

[27] Adapted from Aquinas, T. *Summa Theologica.* Pt. IIa-IIae, Q. 58, Art. 1.

The Unity of the Four Values and Virtues

Human life enjoys a unity in which we are united as brothers and sisters in the human family. A profound implication of this unity of human life is that we are all connected. This fundamental connection implies a brotherhood and sisterhood in the family of humankind. In this light, Citizen Advocacy is one way, among others, to raise the question, "Who is my neighbor?" If we truly believe in the unity of human life, then my neighbor is my brother, my sister.

We all, of course, fall short of this ideal. Yet our interconnectedness as human beings means that what hurts one of us hurts *all* of us, including the most marginal, lowly person among us. What hurts an unborn child hurts all of us. What hurts a 90-year-old widow in a nursing home hurts all of us. What hurts a forgotten man who has lived seventy years in a state institution hurts all of us. What hurts a child with multiple handicaps, a child who cannot see, hear, walk, or talk hurts all of us. What hurts a desperate youth who buys drugs on the street and sleeps under bridges hurts all of us.

No one comes into this world without connection to mother, father, sister and brother, even when those bonds are fractured during the course of life. We build connections in our lives through every relationship we make. Everything we do, in thought, word, or action, affects someone else. There is no such thing as a private act that does not affect other people.

If we are to discover the true meaning of human dignity, the sanctity of human life, love and justice, these values and virtues must be translated into everyday life. The values of human dignity and sanctity of human life are values of being, while the virtues of love and justice are virtues of doing.

The four pillars I have described share a profound interrelationship. Loving one's neighbor and seeking justice are intrinsically related to the sacred dignity with which each human being is endowed. Human dignity is an endowment, not an achievement. Love and justice, then, spring forth from our sacred dignity as human persons as pure water flows from a wellspring whose source is ineffable and eternal. At their source, human dignity, the sanctity of human life, love and justice are one.

CHAPTER SEVENTEEN

Choosing Between the Bad and the Worse: The Story of Walter and Barry

In contrast to the mutual engagement described in most of the stories shared earlier in this book, Walter and Barry's relationship is in one direction — Walter striving to protect Barry — without much from Barry in return. There is no mutuality of friendship, no dialogue or interaction. Walter is an advocate who tries to do what is right for another human being without regard for what he gets out of the relationship, and indeed, without any guarantee of a positive outcome.

Not all Citizen Advocacy stories have storybook endings. Indeed, some of the most powerful lessons come from stories where, in spite of an advocate's best efforts, the protégé's life remains dismal. Sometimes the benefit of a Citizen Advocacy relationship is not so much the good that happened, but preventing worse things that could have happened. Yet even then, much good may develop within people's hearts and souls. Walter knows that goodness, and, he hopes, so does Barry. Following is Walter and Barry's story as told by Walter Kaan.

I have done a lot of different things in my life. When I first left school, I had a business offering mobile discotheques (in the US, that means I was a "disc jockey"). After that I was in nursing. Then I owned a bicycle shop, and later I was painting. After that I began working with computers — which is what I do now. However, there is no precedent in my life for my relationship with Barry. When I met Barry about ten years ago, I was 31, and was on the board of Illawarra Citizen Advocacy (in Wollongong, Australia). Julie Clarke, the coordinator of Illawarra Citizen Advocacy had an office just around the corner from where my brother worked. I met Julie several times, and slowly but surely I was roped onto the board.

Barry, the man for whom I am an advocate, was somehow discovered by Citizen Advocacy (how that happened escapes me), and it looked like he might be railroaded into a nursing home. A crisis came up in Barry's life where he was having a lot of trouble, and it appeared that the social service system and the community was ganging up on him, so it was my role to see that he was fairly represented. He needed someone who really cared to be a voice for him. I became that person.

Barry has an intellectual disability and lived with a foster family as a child. He had a foster sister who looked after him at school, but a lot of the children made fun of him and picked on him. His foster sister tried to protect him and was his only refuge. As Barry grew up he became more competent. Barry worked as an ambulance driver, gaining confidence and skills and he had a valued role. He was a member of a local church in Wollongong and was very active in his church community, working on various committees. He may even have been a deacon, but I'm not sure about that. Barry was well liked, and to an extent was a valued member of his community. However, one of the people from the church I spoke with said that while Barry was loved he was still something of an outsider. She said some people only tolerated him, so I don't think he was fully considered an equal. I think he was regarded as something like a mascot, with an attitude of "We love you, but with limitations."

As Barry got to be in his 50s, his behavior slowly started to deteriorate. He became repetitious and would ramble in conversation. He'd focus on a few favorite things in his life, like having a nice cup of tea. Some people were less tolerant than others, and to them he was a little obnoxious. Barry would wander in conversation and want to have a nice cup of tea and talk about himself in the third person. Instead of saying, "I would like a cup of tea," he would say, "Barry would like a cup of tea." Eventually people at the church did not want him around and they locked him out of the church. They even had someone stand in the front of the church to keep him out. I found this very disheartening. Apart from his foster sister, the church was the one social avenue he had in his life, the one place where he felt accepted, and they locked him out.

Barry lived alone. All he had when I met him was his foster sister whom he only saw occasionally, perhaps once every couple weeks. His sister said Barry was always a bit of a loner. When Barry was alone he felt self-sufficient and for a long time he did fairly well on his own. He was on a disability pension and accounted for his own finances. A caseworker helped him out with things from time to time. After he began to deteriorate, however, he was unable to function as an ambulance driver and lost his job.

As I mentioned, in the beginning of our relationship I was a crisis advocate for Barry. I only expected to be involved for a month or two to get Barry's life settled down and get him safe. I tried to stop him from being railroaded into something that wasn't appropriate for him. When I got involved, it looked like he was going to an "easy-way-out" kind of place, such as a nursing home or institution, without trying to figure out what was going on with him. Barry lived a very private life and refused to let anyone into his house. He wouldn't let anyone help tidy up his place. People who tried to help got turned away at his locked screen door. Barry lived in a housing commission unit, which most people would describe as quite harsh. It was government housing for people in the poverty trap. Barry would slip into his place late at night and lock the door behind him.

From talking with people who knew Barry, I learned that he did not spend a lot of time at home. He had a lot of acquaintances and was often out and about talking with people throughout Wollongong, with shop owners and people like that. There were people in the community who looked out for him, like the shop owners, people at the fire and police stations, and people at the missions and inexpensive places where he could get a bite to eat. People knew him on a first name basis. There were people in the community who tried to help him keep track of his cash, which wasn't plentiful, and they often made sure he had something to eat. The ambulance drivers, shopkeepers, or the firemen might say, "Let's go out to the Chinese restaurant" (or what-not), and they would buy him something in a take-away container. I don't think they were trying to get rid of him — there are ways of getting rid of people so they don't come back, and certainly buying him a meal isn't one of them. So I think people in the community had affection for Barry, especially the ambulance drivers who remembered Barry and loved him.

Things happened in Wollongong that were not pleasant. There were times when he was beaten and sexually abused at the local park. One time he showed up at the mission bleeding after having been raped. The people at the mission were looking after umpteen folks who had lots of needs, so they were not in a position to get more personally involved with Barry. There were some truly wonderful people working at the mission, but they had their work cut out for them just feeding people. Incidentally, the mission was operated by the same church that had locked him out.

However, when I got involved Barry was about to lose his independence. The problem that triggered the crisis was that he would walk out into traffic without looking either way. He was only alive by the grace of God, because he wouldn't think to look to the left or right when crossing the street. According to the people at the Wollongong Mission, this had been going on for a couple of years. Barry was well-known by the people at the mission, and they were concerned about his safety.

When I learned that Barry was in trouble, I tried to learn more about him. I went to the ambulance station and talked to the ambulance drivers and to a few other people there to get an idea of who Barry was. Rather than sending him off to a nursing home, I was hoping to help people get to the bottom of the problems he was having. So I organized for Barry to be evaluated by the Prince of Wales Hospital and Psychology Clinic in Sydney. They have a good reputation for neuropsychology. We were trying to get an idea of what was making Barry deteriorate so rapidly, and to see if there was anything that could be done.

One morning at daybreak, a couple of ambulance guys and the caseworkers and the doctors and I showed up at his apartment. What it amounted to was that when he came out of his house I had to grab him because he was scared. There were a lot of people there, some in uniform, so it was quite a traumatic scene. I asked some of the people he knew and recognized from the mission to come along, and one of the women from the mission went with him to the Prince of Wales Hospital as a friendly face.

When all the tests came back, it turned out that Barry had Alzheimer's disease. Essentially this meant that Barry was on a one-way street — there was no turning back to his former life. Sadly, Barry did wind up in a nursing home. After the assessment at the Prince of Wales Hospital, he was sent to a place up in the hills outside Wollongong, a former consumption (tuberculosis) hospital that was converted into a nursing home. I remember at one of our Citizen Advocacy workshops one of the speakers said that sometimes an advocate has to make a decision between the bad and the worse. Barry got the bad. It would have been worse if he were run over by a truck, or hurt in other ways because of how vulnerable he was living on his own.

It has been a challenge to relate to Barry. Until he was in the nursing home, we didn't relate much, I was just in the background. I tried to relate more to Barry after he was in the hospital. I can't say that I have a sense of who Barry is on the inside. I know he was and is a gentle man. His foster sister said he has always been quiet and gentle. I don't know if that is because he has been bashed back into himself, or whether he always was a gentle person. When he went into the hospital, the nurses thought he was gentle as well; they always said he wouldn't hurt a fly.

Once Barry was in the hospital, I had become his legal guardian mainly to look after his medical care. Once the medical crisis was over, I was still responsible for his care. After a while Barry started to recognize me, and I found myself becoming his long-term advocate. That has been really rewarding for me, and I think for Barry as well. A high point in our relationship was that I was able to get his foster sister involved in his life again. I've tried to get other people who knew Barry to spend time with him, but that has not gone so well.

I often ask myself, "What were the options?" If I were asked if I wanted to go live in a nursing home, the answer is absolutely not. I don't want to interpret Barry's living in a nursing home as being positive in any sense. But when I reflect on the choice between the bad and the worse, I resolved to do what I could in spite of how bad the situation was. I've heard the big stories in Citizen Advocacy, and I have seen first hand stories that had a more positive ending. I would love to be one of those heroes, where everything is shiny and bright where it was once dull and horrid. But that is not always the case, and it hasn't been the case in my relationship with Barry. Things are "less worse" than what they might have been, and while I continue to struggle with that, I am still in Barry's life.

Who knows what worse things might have happened had I not been in Barry's life? He could have been on the streets, or killed under the wheel of a truck. Thus far I have not seen any evidence of abuse in the hospital or nursing home. He is extremely afraid of men. It took a year or so before I could build up some trust. During that year, I chatted with people who knew him, I talked with the nurses, the doctors, the caseworkers, the guardianship board — it was a busy year.

I have learned a great deal through my relationship with Barry. I don't tell many people about our relationship, and I don't think many people would really care or notice. I have become a stronger person from knowing Barry. I have come to see responding to Barry as participating in community. As an advocate, you begin to see yourself as fitting into part of a puzzle, rather than being an isolated individual. By relating to Barry, I found myself relating to the community in a different way. My relationship with Barry has brought out my more serious side. Knowing Barry is very grounding; it has brought me down to earth, sometimes very harshly. I have learned that personal advocacy for a vulnerable person is totally and intimately necessary, especially for people like Barry.

One of the benefits of meeting Barry was that I have met some wonderful people, the likes of which have sometimes reduced me to tears. A phrase that applies here is "People are horrible and dreadful sometimes, but a person, that's not the same thing as people." People have done bad things to Barry, but I have met individual people here and there who just make you cry with how beautiful they are — and that includes Barry. That is something that will stay with me forever. Barry, people at the mission, some of the nurses, and some of the other people I've met through my relationship with Barry have been absolutely wonderful.

When I think of the essence of my relationship with Barry, I think about loneliness. Barry was an extremely lonely guy. I have tried to recognize that, if not solve it. Barry is still in the hospital, and he no longer recognizes me. He does not walk or talk, and he has been immobile the last couple of years. He doesn't ask for a cup of tea anymore. I don't know what I mean to him these days, but I know what he means to me. I love Barry. He is part of my family, and he is in my life for life.

Author's Comments

I have the privilege of knowing Walter Kaan as a friend. During my visits to Australia, Walter and I found much in common in the way we look at the world. We both believe that fidelity and commitment are good things, even though we human beings often fall short of those ideals. We both believe that barring the church doors to an "outcast" is wrong.

The capacity for goodness and truth among like-minded people from all walks of life — and from different countries and cultures — is one of the beautiful things about Citizen Advocacy. The capacity of people who may have a different understanding of the transcendent — that which lies beyond what we can see — to share certain values and truths is something of a mystery. This capacity is expressed through a convergence of truth and goodness. While my understanding of where truth and goodness come from is rooted in my faith, that same truth, that same goodness, can shine in the hearts of people whose under-

standing of where those gifts come from differs from mine. Some thinkers explain this as the natural law, a law that is written in the heart of every human being, and which inspires people to seek the good and avoid evil.

Walter pursued the good on Barry's behalf, and he tried to prevent evil things from happening. While much of Barry's life remains unknown, his reclusiveness may have something to do with protecting himself from further rejection, and from the meanness in the world around him. Unfortunately, the protective walls that Barry erected may have kept out the good as well as the bad. There were people around who wanted to help, but Barry would not let them in.

Most of us have experienced some loneliness in life. However, the totality of rejection that Barry experienced in his life is of a different order. It is a window into the abyss of human suffering. These are dark thoughts, but they represent dark realities. Our human desire to avoid suffering makes us want to avoid suffering people. Walter did not turn away from the reality of Barry's loneliness. While Walter has no magic wand that can miraculously make Barry's life "shiny and bright," terrible things could have happened to Barry if not for Walter's presence, such as violence, rape and death. Yet knowing that worse things could have happened does not remove the harshness of life in a nursing home. Walter has no illusions about that, which is a source of ongoing pain. Walter endures that pain for Barry's sake, and as a result, the small ways of making a difference in Barry's life have great meaning. At the end of the day, Walter may be the only person in the world who truly mourns for Barry.

CHAPTER EIGHTEEN

Loving the Life That is Lived:
The Story of Bonnie and Gary

Like many citizen advocates, Bonnie Schleuter had no idea what she was getting into when she began visiting Gary. In reflecting on how Citizen Advocacy relationships evolve, Tom Kohler uses the analogy of a sailboat in port. Once the boat has left the dock and the sails are up, who knows which way the winds will blow? While one may have a goal and direction, who knows what storms (or calm waters) lie ahead? Following is Bonnie and Gary's story in Bonnie's words.

A friend of mine named Gail suggested that I should consider becoming a citizen advocate. Gail, who was on the board of Grand Island Citizen Advocacy, approached me one evening and said that there was a man named Gary who was from Schuyler, my hometown. Gail said Gary was about my age, and had no family or friends involved in his life. I thought, "You know, I don't want to hear this, because I've never been around a person with a disability."

But Gail had planted this seed, which really annoyed me. I thought, "I think God's probably doing this but I don't want to do this." So I thought about it for a couple of months. It was a long time before I agreed to meet Gary. I talked to my sister, who said, "Well, you know, maybe you should try it." So I called Sherry Cook (the Coordinator of Grand Island Citizen Advocacy) and told her I would meet with her and that we would just talk about it. I was really adamant about not having enough time — the old "time" thing. I had time for coffee and lunch and shopping or whatever — but not for this. So we met, and I said, "I'll go see him, but I'm not going to spend a lot of time with him. I'm a busy woman."

Sherry and I went to meet Gary about a week later. He was not being taken care of very well; I could see that right away. He was not open to people approaching him. I'm sure he looked at me and thought, "Who is this woman? Probably someone who is going to breeze in and breeze out." He was a mess, long hair, long nails, not clean — just not taken care of. I don't know what I said to him; I guess I said something, but he was not responding. We took Gary across the street to have a Coke, and then we took him back to the nursing home. When Sherry and I left him and got out into the parking lot, we both immediately burst into tears. That was my first visit.

The next time I went back, I went alone. I was brave. I had no idea what I was going to do. I took a candy bar and a Coke, and we sat in Gary's room and talked. I noticed he didn't have anything personal in his room except some black and white pictures from when he was growing up. So we talked about that. Gary could talk but it was hard to understand him. He couldn't hear, so his speech wasn't the best. I probably stayed maybe twenty minutes, which felt like a long time. I visited him a couple times that first week.

The next week I went back three times. Then the next week I went back every day, and the next thing I was going on weekends. I didn't stay a long time, but I always told him I'd be back and what time. I knew he probably didn't trust me, and maybe he didn't trust anything that anybody told him, so I knew telling him when I'd be back was important. It got to be where I had to see him every day just to make sure that he was okay. He wasn't well cared for at all. My primary goal was to ensure that he got better care.

It took a couple of months, maybe longer, to win his trust. I knew

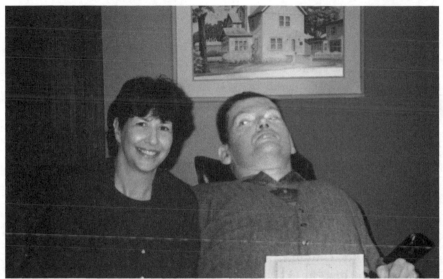

Bonnie and Gary

he was tolerating my visits, but I wasn't quite sure what he thought about me. I'd ask him and he would look at me, but I couldn't tell what he was thinking. I knew he liked soft drinks and candy. We would go for walks around the nursing home. It was July, so it was hot. Gary's skin was pasty white, and he had never been outside — at least not for a long time, maybe even years. He never got to do anything. So I thought, "We'll just go for a little walk and get him out." He seemed to enjoy that. We'd go sit out on the patio, outside of the facility, because he never left his room except for meals.

Gary lived there for almost twenty years. I think he got a bath once a week. They maybe shaved him once a week. His nails were long. He had hair growing out of his nose and ears, and his skin was white and scaly. His lips were chapped. These were simple little things, things that should have been taken care of to make him feel better. His shirt would be open, they never snapped it, they just threw it on, and so his shirt would hang off his shoulders. That was hard for me. It made me angry that no one could see the obvious. There were flies in his room and Gary couldn't move, so there would be flies landing on him. Things we take for granted, like itching our noses, or swatting a fly, taking a drink of water, these were

211

things he couldn't do. It must have been maddening and over-whelming for Gary to have to go for hours without even the most basic kinds of care and attention.

I knew I had to start by gaining his trust. I had to let him know that I would always come back and that he could count on me. Gradually, I worked on his grooming. I shaved him, trimmed his nails, and made sure he got a haircut. He couldn't have felt good about his appearance looking like he did — how could he? I brought him some cologne and some new clothes so that he could see other ways to be and feel. Later on, we started going into town. One of the first things we did was go out and have coffee. But in a nursing home you just can't say, "Okay we're going out now." You have to ask the nurses, you have to plan it, and they have to have the van available. Gary couldn't transfer into a car because he had to be lying back or else he couldn't breathe. He had to be in a certain position, like in a recliner chair, so he could breathe. He would have loved riding in a car, because he sat so high in the van that he couldn't see well.

We walked about a mile to the radio station where I worked and had a tour. He was a big guy, so that wasn't easy. One time the wheelchair got stuck on the railroad tracks when we were going to the grocery store. He was stuck on the tracks, and I got scared and found all this strength and got him out. I don't know if he realized we were in trouble, which was probably good.

We would talk about where to go. I'd say, "You know I won't take you anyplace where you'll be uncomfortable," or, "We'll go for an hour." He needed to know that I would never let anything bad hap-pen. People would stare at us; he was very brave to go out. But a lot of people came up and talked to him — he really liked that. They thought I was either his sister or his wife, or some kind of rel-ative, because they thought, "Who would actually do this?" I'd say, "I'm an advocate." They'd say, "What's an advocate?" People are so surprised that you could become involved on a freely-given basis and do this for somebody — which is kind of sad in and of itself.

Some of the nursing staff really liked me, but others hated me, because I made them do their job. If he was sick or needed some-thing, I wanted it taken care of. I didn't want him denied. I called one of the nurses "Nurse Ratchet;"[28] she hated me. They had to give him better care because they knew I was coming — at any given time, on any given day. Like anywhere else, if you have a friend or a family member checking on you, you're going to get better care. They got so used to Gary just sitting in his room and not having to do anything but feed him, my being around and asking questions meant more work for them. Although, I did a lot of things for Gary. I shaved him and did a lot of grooming things. I helped clean his room and things like that. If they could have seen it this way, I was really an asset.

One of the nurses, a nursing supervisor, was really a nice girl. One time she called to tell me they were taking him to the hospital. Gary had a fever, and I was upset. She said, "I didn't know if I should call you or not, because I knew you'd get emotional." I said, "I love him, of course I'm going to get emotional. Who needs to be there more than me?" I thought that was strange. I know that nurses can't get emotional with every person because so many people die there, and they don't want to get attached, but that's no excuse for not identifying with people. If this were my brother, son or spouse, how would I feel? . . .

There were also some funny things that happened. Gary's roommate had a black and white TV. He was in a big room with three other men and the TV was in the back. He would watch cartoons on the black and white TV, or it would be fuzzy. So I wanted to buy him a new TV. I had given him a used color TV, but it didn't work very well. I wanted him to use some of his own money to buy a TV. He had several thousand dollars that he needed to use or it would go back to the state. I tried to explain this to him, but he said, "No spend money, no TV." So I said, "Okay, here's the deal, let's just get a TV and try it. If you don't like it, I'll take it back." So we got this color TV and set up a remote. I don't remember how we did it, but we used Velcro and a lot of superglue. He had a tray, and I used Velcro to put the remote on the tray, and then I put little Velcro

---

[28] Nurse Ratchet refers to a character in a book by Ken Kesey, later made into a movie entitled, "One Flew Over The Cuckoo's Nest," who is a controlling, mean, hateful head nurse in a psychiatric state hospital set in the 1950s.

pieces on the remote channels. He couldn't turn to the channels, but he could run up and down the channels and turn it on or off. Who knows how long it had been since he was able to control his own TV. He thought that was pretty cool. He could move his finger and turn his TV on and off. He was pretty pleased. That was probably his first real freedom, just having that. My husband, whose name is also Gary, bought an entertainment center for Gary's TV and stereo. That caused quite a stir. People would come in and say, "Look at your entertainment center!" We also got him moved to a different room. There were so many changes in his life; I should have kept a diary, but you know it's just life and you just do it — you don't think about it.

A lot of things I did with Gary were just simple things, and often, funny things. One day I was trying to talk him into doing something, and he mumbled something and I knew he was mad. I said, "You're mad." He shook his head "No," because being angry was not acceptable to him. I said, "Well, it's okay to get mad at me, you can get mad at me. Let's talk about this." Then he quieted down, and I said, "It's okay." I'm sure sometimes he thought, "Where did this woman come from? How long do I have to put up with her?"

Another time I was trying to make him more comfortable by putting his feet up on the wheelchair pads to lessen the pressure, and he was mumbling under his breath — he wasn't cooperating. I said, "Work with me here, Gar, work with me." It was just hysterical. Some of the things I'd say, he'd just look at me as if to say, "What are you talking about?"

Gary liked to smoke; he hadn't smoked for years, but he wanted to smoke a cigarette. After a while, I was beginning to understand him better, and he told me he wanted a cigarette. He got a hearing aid, and that helped. So I said, "I can bring you cigarettes, we can do this." The nurse said, "I don't think the doctor wants him to smoke." I said, "Well I don't think it's any of the doctor's business." So we would go out on the patio and have a Coke and we'd smoke. He wouldn't inhale. We did that maybe three times a week, which I didn't think was going to kill anybody. One day he must have seen something on TV that smoking causes cancer. I asked him, "Do you want to go have a cigarette?" He said, "No." I asked why, and he said, "Dander," or at least that's what I thought he said. I said, "Spell it." He said, "c-a-n-c-e-r". And I said, "Oh, cancer. Honey, you won't get cancer from smoking three cigarettes a week." He never smoked after that.

We tried to vote. Actually, we did vote. Trying to read some of those amendments was funny. I'd say, "I don't know what this means; I don't know what to do." So we'd vote on the things I understood. I would have loved to have read his mind just to see what he was thinking about my explanation of the amendments.

Gary came to our house one day for a visit. I live in an old house, and it was hard to get him in. But my husband Gary was going to get him in the house, even if he had to tear the top of the door off. My daughter Aubrey and Gary bonded right away. What took me six months to do, it took Aubrey maybe ten minutes. Gary really liked her; she was so natural with him. She loved him. My family learned a lot from being with Gary; it was a learning experience. My friends had never been exposed to people with disabilities, just like me, but then they'd go to the nursing home to see Gary. They would ask if they could do things for him. If I was away I always had somebody check on him. He got a lot of love and care in a short amount of time.

We needed each other. I needed to learn patience, of which I have none. I didn't know I could love him so much. It's not like you love your children, or your husband; it's different. I have friends who I love, but this love was almost fierce. He had a nurse who abused him at the nursing home — this was before he met me. I probably would have killed her, and we'd be doing this [interview] in jail. She was a mean, big, nurse who abuses everybody in her care, not just Gary, but Gary was an easy target. One night she was shaving him and he didn't want her to. Gary didn't like her, and so she shaved part of his head. They pulled her off the floor, so she's abusing other patients. I would watch and make sure that she wasn't on his floor. A couple times she was on his floor, and I would say to him, "You know, I want to know." I would ask him, "Has she been in here? Has she done anything? I want you to tell me." I don't think she did anything because by then she knew I was around. We were going to a Citizen Advocacy annual dinner one night, and she drove us. We got him all dressed up that night, got him some new clothes, and I said, "Let's have a date." We put him in the van and I got him belted in; I think she would have just shoved him in the back of the van not belted to anything. I got him all belted in and sat in the front seat. While we were driving, I said, "You know, Gary and I have a really good relationship. He tells me everything that happens at the nursing home." As she drove, I said, "You know, he just tells me everything." I thought, "If that doesn't take care of it, we'll do something else, but I want you to know that I know about you." . . .

Gary always had a fever, but they could never figure out what it was. Nothing seemed to help. The last six months of his life he was in the hospital three times. He had a "Do Not Resuscitate" (DNR) order on his chart, so sometimes they would question, "do we take him (to the hospital) or do we not?" It was hard. Sometimes he would stop breathing. I think his body was worn out. I talked to him about the DNR. I think the nursing home just assumed that there should be a DNR. I remember saying to him, "You know, if something happens to you, do you want to die, or do you want to go to the hospital?" Well, Gary hated hospitals. Regardless of whether he wanted to die or not, he would not choose to go to the hospital.

I wanted him to stay alive. I wanted him to stay alive because I wanted him to, not because he wanted to. I just wanted him to have as good a life as he could while he was here. I wanted him to know that he could have a better life and that he was loved. The bottom line is that he was loved. I would say to him, "I love you." Then I'd say, "I know you love me." He would never say it, but he would blink. I would say, "I will never let anybody hurt you." He knew that; he knew he was loved.

I'm surprised Gary lived as long as he did. I know he got better care after I became involved. I don't know if he wanted his life extended or not, but as long as I was in it, he was going to get all the care he could get. I know he got better care at the hospital. One time they called me from the nursing home and said the ambulance took Gary to the hospital. I rushed down to the hospital and he was in the emergency room, and at first they would not let me see him because I'm not family. They said, "Who are you?" I said, "I'm his advocate." Well, nobody understands what that is, so I go through this little dance, "I'm his friend, I take care of him, I'm like family but I'm not." I said to the lady in charge, "I'm *better* than family, okay, so you *better* let me in." After that, they let me back to see him. He was in the emergency room for quite a while. I guess that's normal, but it made Gary uncomfortable. I told the nurses what makes him comfortable, that he couldn't talk, that he needed to be elevated, that his legs needed pillows — things that he can't communicate. Plus he was scared and burning up with fever. I got him settled for the night and he stayed two or three days. I had to make sure they gave him enough liquids, because he can't drink without help. He needed someone there to say, "This is what he needs; call me if he needs something."

One of the other times he was in the emergency room I found him in one of the cubicles, yelling. He was mad — he hardly ever yelled. A nurse was trying to draw blood from his arm, but Gary's veins were so thin because he had poor circulation. The nurse was digging around in his arm, and he was angry. If he could have hit her I think he would have; he was really upset. I didn't even go to the front desk. I just walked in, went back there and said to the nurse, "You need to not do this right now, I need to talk to Gary." She didn't say to him, "I know this hurts, I know this is hard." She was just taking his blood, without trying to help him through it. So we got through that and he was admitted in the morning. By 3:00 in the afternoon he still had not had lunch, and the doctor hadn't ordered anything. So I went to the nurse and said, "Okay, here's the deal, he needs some soup, he needs some Jell-O, he needs some beverages, and he needs some medication, and I want it done now." The nurse said, "We don't have orders from the doctor." I said, "Call him." Within fifteen minutes we had food. No other person would have been treated that way. That isn't right. When you're disabled, they just put you in a room to wait until they're good and ready, almost as if they had forgotten him.

One time I had to go out of town for three or four days, so I had people check on him — people he knew. People would go see him, and he would shake his head or blink his eyes, which was his way of showing that he accepted them. I wanted him to know he was loved and protected. He wouldn't let me do a lot of things, but we made his room better and did what we could to make him more comfortable. If I could have brought him home, I would have. He would have lived with me, but he needed too much care. We talked about him living on his own, but that was scary to him. . . .

Gary died on a Friday. I was out of town visiting my mother-in-law in a nursing home. I got back late, about 5:30 or 6:00 PM. I had called because I told Gary I would come by. I called the nursing home and said I was really tired, and please tell Gary I will be there in the morning. He died at suppertime.

One of the nurses came to the house to tell me, which was really nice. It was about 8:30 at night, and she came over and got me — they were very good about it. I got to go sit with him in his room. I was probably there a couple of hours. I talked to him. I had some friends come over and some of the nursing staff came in and checked on me — the ones who liked Gary and me. I got to spend time with him the next day. He was here in town. Then we went to Schuyler to the funeral home to spend time with him. My daughter came, and two friends of Gary's came. We laughed, we cried, we said goodbye. His heart just stopped, which is what they said would probably happen. They tried to resuscitate him, but it was just his time. We had a funeral planned for him; we personalized it. It was a little uncomfortable, because his family was pretty closed. I brought pictures. Four of us got up and shared about the Gary we knew. I felt a little selfish, because I was saying things his own family didn't know, but I wanted his family to know that Gary was loved. He had a better life. I had mixed feelings, like I was stepping on toes, but Gary deserved this. Maybe his family got to understand a little bit of what Gary was really like. We laughed and told stories. I guess it was just one of those things where you don't quite know what you're going to do until you get there. He knew he was loved. That was the best thing.

Who could have known? I mean, what a relationship. You take a man who rarely spoke and never had much life experience and was so secluded, and then you take me — no patience, no experience, no plan for what to do with Gary — and it turns out to be a perfect match. Who would have thought he would let me into his life? He didn't have any reason to trust me or to love me. I know God must have been in this, because this isn't anything I could have figured out.

Author's Comments

When Citizen Advocacy was first conceptualized, many people claimed that ordinary citizens would not make lasting personal commitments to people with disabilities. Since Bonnie was not a family member, some claimed she had no legitimate voice in Gary's life. For vulnerable people who do not have family, or if what family they do have is not involved, this is a dangerous assumption. In many human service facilities, people who do not have a committed ally essentially become the "property" of the service delivery system, and as property, they may be treated or mistreated as the service provider sees fit. Bonnie's consistent presence gave her standing in Gary's life, which enabled her to protect Gary from harm.

Gary was not used to making decisions for himself, and probably did not have many opportunities to learn how to make decisions. Decisions that have life and death implications, such as whether or not to go to the hospital, or whether or not to have a "do not resuscitate" (DNR) order, must be examined in light of Gary's past experiences. Gary had reasonable fears about hospitals, and he had some terrible experiences in emergency rooms. Why would he opt to go to a hospital if he could avoid it? Gary was probably unaware that for socially devalued people, DNR orders are often interpreted as "do not treat" orders. Even simple procedures or treatments may be withheld for people who have DNRs, especially people like Gary who some people might consider as not having a life worth living.

In medical circles, "autonomy" — what the patient says he wants — is presumed to carry a lot of weight. However, some "decisions" are not really decisions at all, but programmed responses influenced by previous life experiences. When a person's life is at stake, and that person makes decisions that are dangerous to life or limb, someone needs to challenge that person's "decision." Life is more important than autonomy, and one cannot very well exercise one's autonomy when one is dead.

One will not find the profound, inexplicable love that Bonnie and Gary shared in every Citizen Advocacy relationship, nor should one expect to. Some relationships are based more on a sense of justice rather than love. In other relationships, like Bonnie and Gary's, justice and love are united.

When I visited Bonnie in Nebraska for this interview, John Murphy, the Citizen Advocacy support person from Nebraska Advocacy Services, took me on a personal tour of Lincoln. On the campus of the University of Nebraska there is a bronze sculpture of a man lying on his deathbed, apparently having recently died. Integral to the sculpture is a figure of a woman — perhaps his wife or daughter — stretched out over his legs in a posture of deep sorrow, overwhelmed with grief. The man is dressed in simple clothing, probably a farmer. He has a beatific smile on his face, the smile of a man who died in peace. The woman is folded into the figure of the man in a way that makes her sorrow and his peace as one. The beauty of the man's expression and the depth of the woman's sorrow in one image are, in a word, stunning.

As I reflected on that image, I thought of Bonnie and Gary. To die without love, without having at least one person in the world whose heart is broken by grief, is the ultimate loneliness. Gary did not die such a death. He knew he was loved, with a love that overcomes death.

When I interviewed Bonnie I was trying to learn the lessons of life-protecting Citizen Advocacy relationships. The most important lesson I came away with was not about life-protecting strategies — however important such strategies might be. What I realized instead is that protecting a person's life is more about loving the life that is lived, rather *than about "how-to" strategies for defending a person's life. Bonnie wanted Gary to live because she loved him. It was her love, not abstract ideas about the value of life, which moved her to protect Gary's life.*

This is not to say that abstract ideas — especially ideas about the value of life — are not important. They are. Ideas have consequences, and the idea that human life is precious is certainly an idea that should motivate a person to defend another person's life. We are more than our ideas, however, and for Bonnie, it was her love, rather than concepts about the value of a person's life, that inspired her actions. Bonnie helped Gary live a fuller life, as well as a longer life, because she loved him.

AFTERWORD

In Citizen Advocacy, we see much joy and laughter. I sometimes worry that I have focused too much on the valleys — on the woundedness of people's lives. I want to focus more on the lighter side of life, and speak more of the joys of Citizen Advocacy relationships, because those are uplifting, and they are real. Yet I am compelled to speak of the hard parts of life that so many of us deny or avoid. It is possible that I may have characterized the life experiences of devalued people in a way that leaves the impression that wounds are all there is to people. All people, without exception, bear some wounds in life. Whether one is wounded by virtue of our birth into an imperfect world, or wounded by the slings and arrows of life's misfortunes, we are all, as one ancient writer put it, "born into this vale of tears." That is part and parcel of the human condition. In my worldview, I believe we are born with a wound in our soul, so to speak, and that the purpose of this life is the healing of that wound. If knowing that we are all wounded can foster a deeper awareness of our human limitations — and through that awareness, humility — perhaps we can better relate to devalued people whose wounds may be more obvious.

Over the years, we have seen much suffering in Citizen Advocacy. I remember a man curled up in his bed, blind, and paralyzed, who had not had a visitor for over four years; the young man with autism who had been sexually abused by his father, so frightened that he hadn't left his apartment for more than 20 years; the young woman who seemed destined to live out the rest of her life in a nursing home; the young man whose life was turned upside down by a severe neck injury, and who died because they removed his feeding tube. Once we met a young man with a mild mental handicap, and as we sat with him and his mom in their kitchen, he put his head on his mother's shoulder, sobbing, saying, "I wish I wasn't born like this." I could go on.

For most people, reconciling oneself to suffering in the world takes a lifetime. If we are not able to deal with our own suffering, we will hardly be able to deal with, or even recognize, the suffering we encounter in the lives of people around us. Only when we find meaning in suffering can we become reconciled to the suffering of people in the larger community and in the wider world.

Life does not lose its preciousness when life gets hard. If life has inherent meaning, then *all* of life must have inherent meaning. Therefore suffering, as much as one would wish to avoid it, has meaning. Why some people suffer more than others, and why innocent children suffer, is an unfathomable mystery for which there simply is no answer in this life.

I believe that the only way to adaptively cope with suffering is to *embrace* it. By embracing suffering, I do not mean that one should love to suffer, but that one should love the sufferer. To embrace suffering means to open oneself up, heart, mind and soul to another person's suffering. Yes, there is much we can do to prevent suffering, to minimize it, and to compensate for it, but at the end of the day, we will not be able to get rid of human suffering. We are only human, and suffering will always be with us, at least in this life.

Embracing suffering is the secret to real joy in life. As Kahlil Gibran said, "The more that sorrow carves into your heart, the more joy it can contain."[29] It is when we join suffering to sacrificial love — a pure giving of self — that real joy can enter our lives. For one to experience true joy, a joy that will last, one must be close to, and stay close to, suffering people. Standing with someone who is hurting keeps one's feet on the ground. It teaches us and shows us what is real. The most profound moments of your life have probably included either love or suffering or both. Mountaintop experi-

---

[29] Gibran, K. (1972). *The Prophet*. New York: Alfred A. Knopf, Inc. p. 29.

ences in our lives, those peaks of human existence, happen when love and suffering are united in a transcendent joy — something that words cannot describe. Some readers may be yet too young to hear and understand these words, but life will someday teach you this lesson, if you are open to it.

It is our woundedness that gives us the capacity to live in community with one another. When we open our hearts to a wounded person, we open ourselves up to the possibility of being hurt. When we expose our vulnerabilities, we take the chance that someone will take advantage of our weakness. Yet in our vulnerability, we find our greatest strength, and our attempt to maintain a strong invincible posture to the world around us is the very thing that prevents us from finding a source of healing deep within the human heart.

Recognizing our vulnerability as human beings uproots human pride and tears down barriers to genuine human relationship. Once this discovery is made, we are then able to see others as ourselves. A citizen advocate in Georgia gave me a glimpse of what this means. The advocate had helped a young man with mental retardation find and furnish an apartment, get a job, and establish a life in the community. I asked her why she did what she did, and why she continues to stand by this young man. Her answer was clear and direct. She said, "I look at him as if he were me, and then I help him."

Citizen Advocacy gives people the opportunity to be moved by compassion — to be moved in their hearts. It lifts the veil of assumptions, stereotypes and prejudice to help a citizen see a neighbor with a disability as a person, a human being whose life has inherent, intrinsic, precious and absolute worth and dignity.

Human history is replete with efforts to make the world a better place, to establish or find utopia. "Utopia" literally means "no place on earth." Any serious review of human history easily demonstrates that all efforts to establish utopia have failed. When we look at our failures, it is easier to point the finger at "the system," or at other people, rather than at ourselves. We do not want to recognize or admit our own individual human failings.

My realization that the world we live in will never be perfect has come more from a realization that I will never be perfect. Some decades ago, an essay contest was held on the question: "What is wrong with the world?" One writer, G.K. Chesterton, submitted his essay consisting of two words, "I am."

Yet there is hope. It is in and through our woundedness that a light can begin to shine. When we discover our vulnerabilities, we realize the folly of thinking more of ourselves than others. When we see a wounded person as someone who offers an opportunity for healing of our own wounds, there is hope. Jean Vanier has said, "This is the mystery: those who appear to be less human teach us to be more human, and those who are most rejected are those who heal us."[30]

The citizen advocates I know in Beaver, Pennsylvania, and the citizen advocates I have met in other parts of the world, give me great hope. Hope has little to do with reason. Hope springs from deep within the human heart, from a place where a person desires a better tomorrow. By hope, I do not mean a simple optimistic outlook, or a "think good thoughts" mind-set, or even a hope that relies on positive outcomes. Hope is an expectation of something desired, something better than what is now — something that ought to be. I hope that the Citizen Advocacy movement will continue to find advocates, one person at a time, time after time.

Citizen Advocacy is personal, and so I conclude with a personal reflection. Writing these words on a cold January morning, I am sitting in my boyhood home, looking out the window. Snowflakes drift and swirl about, the evergreens laden with snow. I think of beautiful times in my life, warm and safe against the evils in the world, the bitter cold a contrast to the warmth of my childhood memories. I recall my father's singing, my mother's pancakes, building snowmen, hot chocolate after sled-riding.

Then I remember a woman whose voice I hear when I visit our local nursing home. She cries, "Nurse, where am I?" her eyes swollen with tears. I see a young man in his wheelchair, head bent low, sitting in the midst of trash strewn about his apartment, his

---

[30] De Souza, R.J. Vanier speaks on the "handicapped" Pope for lent. *National Catholic Register,* February 17-23, 2002, p. 5.

mother angry at the world. A smell of filth makes me afraid to touch anything. I think of orphaned children living in sewers in China, African children dying from AIDS, and countless people in nursing homes, boarding homes, and other places for abandoned people, sitting, waiting to die.

How do these, how can these, two worlds co-exist? How can the world of beauty and of love, of Christmas carols and hot chocolate, and the world of brokenness, of suffering, of despair, and of death exist in the same time and place? How is it, and why is it, that I live a privileged life, while only miles or even blocks away, so many people live lives of quiet desperation?

I have had suffering in my life — the death of my father and my brother, personal losses and failures, and a pervasive melancholy that seems ever poised to steal my joy. Yet in balance, my life is one of many blessings — of children, of friends, of opportunities to make a difference in the world. I am further blessed by a taste of suffering in my life that enables me to hear the cries of the oppressed. Their suffering, while far greater than my own, speaks to my wounds in life. Had I not known suffering, I would not hear their voices. Yet I struggle to keep my eyes open, my ears hearing, and my heart feeling. I grow weary of listening to the groans of hurting people and want to turn away. I want to close my eyes, block my ears, protect my heart. . . . But I fear that if I do that, my heart will grow cold. A cold heart does not feel pain or joy. A cold heart does not feel anything at all.

My work over the past 16 years in Citizen Advocacy has been to ask people to look at what they see, listen to what they hear, and move when their hearts are moved. In the end, asking people to open their hearts is both the destination and the journey.

APPENDIX A

An orientation to Citizen Advocacy Principles

Citizen Advocacy is guided by a number of core ideas or principles that clarify and safeguard independent advocacy by citizens on behalf of vulnerable people. Briefly stated, these principles are:

Advocate Independence
Citizen advocates engage in a freely-given, freely-chosen, relationship. Citizen advocates are independent of human services, the protégé's family, and of the Citizen Advocacy office itself.

Loyalty to Protégé
The primary loyalty of a citizen advocate is to his protégé. An advocate's actions are based on his understanding of the protégé.

Program Independence
The Citizen Advocacy organization is independent of service providing agencies, and of other advocacy forms. Citizen Advocacy finds its identity and support from within the broader community, not the human service system.

Clarity of Staff Function
The role of the Citizen Advocacy program staff is to recruit and support citizen advocates, not to be advocates themselves, or to engage

in other forms of advocacy.

Diversity of Relationships
A Citizen Advocacy program recruits advocates for people who have a wide range of identities and needs, and so citizen advocates fill a wide range of flexible roles.

Positive Imagery
Citizen Advocacy strives to counter the negative images so commonly associated with devalued people by promoting positive, dignifying images in whatever ways possible.

Before giving a more in-depth explanation of these principles, it may help to clarify what a principle is, and how effective implementation of the Citizen Advocacy principles can benefit individual citizen advocates. When an architect designs a house, he applies certain design principles that guide the builders in such a way as to prevent the roof from caving in, keep water from leaking in the basement, maximize living space, create a comfortable environment, and so on. If the architect chooses to ignore the basic design principles for building a house, he does so at considerable risk to the people who buy the house. A good architect knows that design principles are not just some autocratic set of ideas that someone arbitrarily thought up. The principles for the design of houses were crafted from experience. The authors of architectural design principles learned from the mistakes of people whose houses did not stand because of poor design. They also based their principles on what was found to be effective in the building of a solid house that will withstand the elements over time.

Similarly, the architects of Citizen Advocacy were well-informed about advocacy design, both from their own experiences and from the experiences of others. Wolfensberger examined the variety of protection and advocacy forms in existence at the time, and sought to combine the best elements of advocacy while avoiding common pitfalls in advocacy. While the principles of advocacy design may not be as observable as blueprints for a house, they are no less real. Wolfensberger sought to design a form of advocacy that was:

a. Minimizing of conflicts of interests;

b. Flexible according to the individual identities and needs of protégés;

c. Designed to incorporate personal, individualized one-to-one (or near one-to-one) relationships; and

d. Supported by a competent Citizen Advocacy office that was itself free of conflicts of interests.

Citizen advocates benefit from careful and effective implementation of the Citizen Advocacy principles in many ways. For example, a citizen advocate's primary loyalty to the protégé makes it clear that the advocate is free (and expected) to act according to what he or she sees as most relevant for his protégé. An independent Citizen Advocacy program is less likely to be pressured to control an advocate or to water down what an advocate is asked to do for fear of retribution. Clarity about the role of Citizen Advocacy staff helps a program coordinator to avoid taking over the role of a citizen advocate. These are just a few of the concrete ways in which advocates — and protégés — benefit from careful implementation of the Citizen Advocacy principles. Following is a more detailed discussion of issues that Citizen Advocacy programs commonly encounter as they implement the principles of Citizen Advocacy.

Advocate Independence

Citizen advocates engage in a freely-given, freely-chosen, relationship. Citizen advocates are independent of human services, a protégé's family, and of the Citizen Advocacy office itself.

The Nebraska state capitol building has the following quote etched in marble above its main entrance: "The health of the state is dependent on the watchfulness of its citizens." On a person-to-person level, Citizen Advocacy relies on the watchfulness of individual citizens who will promote justice for vulnerable people. To be truly watchful and vigilant, citizen advocates must be independent. Citizen Advocacy puts its trust in competent, valued, independent citizens who are not afraid to speak up and be heard.

People with disabilities and other devalued people often have a variety of people and organizations that exert great influence over their lives, such as family members, service providers, or even friends. The reason why advocate independence is so important is that there are always some competing interests in any given situation. A conflict of interest does not necessarily mean that one person's interests are valid and another person's interests invalid, or that one person is good and the other bad. Two parties may both have legitimate interests that compete with one another.

For example, a residential service provider has an interest in providing a service at a reasonable cost so as to stay within an agency budget, and yet one or several of its residents may need extra support beyond what the agency can afford. Another example is that agencies have an interest in protecting their reputations, so incidents of abuse or neglect by a service-providing agency might not receive public attention. Advocates need to be aware of such conflicts, and promote the interests of the protégé when those interests are at risk of being compromised. It is therefore important that advocates be independent of the agencies and service providers who have controlling interests in the lives of protégés.

Another feature of advocate independence is that advocates are independent of the protégé's family and friends. This kind of independence sounds counterintuitive, as the province of family responsibility towards vulnerable family members is almost sacred ground. However, not all families in all circumstances or at all times act in the best interests of a vulnerable family member. Being independent of the interests of a protégé's family (or of a service provider) does not necessarily mean that an advocate has to have an adversarial relationship with them. When a family does have the best interests of its family member at heart, an advocate can represent the interests of his protégé in ways that help the protégé's perspective to be seen and heard. Sometimes it takes an "outsider" to help the family see the protégé's point of view. This does not necessarily mean that a family is ill-intentioned; it simply means that the dynamics of family life are almost always complicated.

For example, a family member may be exhausted from keeping vigil at a hospital or nursing home and needs to get some rest — which competes with the protégé's need for someone at the bedside. A more worrisome example is when a distraught family member of someone with complex medical needs might regard a person who is suffering as "better off dead." A family member may even say something to that effect, although the words uttered in such situations are rarely so stark. One may instead hear phrases like "low quality of life" or "she would not have wanted to live this way." In our present medical culture, such words are sometimes used to justify inappropriately withholding or withdrawing needed treatment or even food and water. Most conflicts of interests in families are not so dramatic, and may involve what freedoms a person is allowed, or how someone's money is handled, planning (or lack of it) for the future, and other concerns that fall within the domain of family life.

A word of caution: families have always been — and for most people will continue to be — a primary source of support. An advocate needs to tread lightly before interfering in a family's business, but there are times when someone outside the family needs to raise a voice on a person's behalf. Ideally, this is done by someone who has relevant standing in a person's life — an advocate whose relationship is tried and true.

The independence of advocates means that advocates have the freedom, and the responsibility, to decide whether or not to become an advocate, what they will do, and when they will do it. However, advocate independence does not mean that advocates are left on their own without support. Citizen advocates should be able to rely on competent, knowledgeable advice from their local Citizen Advocacy office, and at the same time be free to make their own independent judgments. I have often said to advocates, "I will offer you advice provided that you feel free not to take it." Supporting an advocate while respecting and preserving the advocate's independence involves walking a fine line between "managing" a relationship and offering — but not imposing — relevant support to an advocate.

Loyalty to Protégé

The primary loyalty of a citizen advocate is to his protégé. An advocate's actions are based on his understanding of the protégé.

An easy way for a citizen advocate to understand this principle is to ask herself, "Who am I really here for?" The answer, of course, is the protégé. However, acting on this principle can often be confused and compromised by other loyalties. An advocate from time to time may need to remind herself, or have others remind her (such as a Citizen Advocacy coordinator), that her first concern is the protégé. To keep this focus, and advocate must look at the world through the eyes of her protégé.

The primary loyalty of an advocate to a protégé is largely influenced by the extent to which an advocate identifies with the protégé. Identification prompts an advocate to ask questions like: "How would I feel if I had to live here, eat this food, sleep in this bed, deal with this human service worker? What would I be thinking and feeling if this person were my son or daughter, my mother or father, my sister or brother? What would I want for my life if I were in this person's shoes?" The best way, and perhaps the only way, for an advocate to maintain a clear primary loyalty to the protégé is to constantly strive to see things from the protégé's perspective.

Advocates often find themselves developing loyalties to other people in their protégé's life, especially to family members, and sometimes, to likeable and/or influential human service workers. Developing loyalties to individual human service workers is particularly troublesome, as conflicts of interests posed by service delivery systems will almost always mean that the interests of the more powerful party — the service system — will prevail. Loyalties to families are more understandable, but an advocate must still keep his primary loyalty to the protégé clearly in focus. Even loving, caring people can do things that are hurtful. Making prudential judgments about such situations is a delicate matter, and calls for wise counsel and support. For citizen advocates, this may come from the Citizen Advocacy office, or from other trusted people who possess such wisdom.

Program Independence

The Citizen Advocacy organization is independent of service providing agencies, and of other advocacy forms. Citizen Advocacy finds its identity and support from within the broader community, not the human service system.

Just as the idea of each citizen advocate acting on his own volition, is important, so is the idea of the Citizen Advocacy program being independent. Citizen Advocacy programs should see themselves as freestanding enterprises. This is different from having, for example, a mentoring program that is the volunteer component of a deinstitutionalization plan, or the provider of volunteers for people living at the local institution or nursing home.

A Citizen Advocacy organization needs to have its own identity, mission, and strategies for action. Citizen Advocacy programs must make decisions about who they find advocates for, who they find as advocates, what they ask advocates to do, and how they support advocates. The Citizen Advocacy staff must be free to develop their own understanding of who potential protégé's are, and to help advocates discern positive futures for protégés.

Program independence has implications for the location of the office, the identity of the staff, the governance of the organization, and the sources of financial support upon which a Citizen Advocacy program relies. Some funding sources have strings attached that compromise Citizen Advocacy. Program independence usually depends on a diversity of funding sources independent of human service funding. Most Citizen Advocacy organizations strive to sustain themselves through a combination of local grass-roots support, private philanthropy, and government sources not directly tied to local service provision.

Clarity of Staff Function

The role of the Citizen Advocacy program staff is to recruit and support citizen advocates, not to be advocates themselves, or to engage in other forms of advocacy.

Useful maxims for focused, effective action are: "Be what you are" and "Do what you do." A citizen advocacy coordinator is a person who makes matches and supports Citizen Advocacy relationships. As such, what a Citizen Advocacy coordinator *does* is — make matches and support relationships. This is so easy to say, and yet keeping one's focus on making matches and supporting relationships is difficult.

The difficulty lies in the fact that coordinating a Citizen Advocacy enterprise involves a complex set of tasks that require high energy and intense focus. A Citizen Advocacy coordinator can easily get caught up in producing newsletters, raising money, giving presentations, devising elaborate filing systems, "networking," and anything and everything besides making matches and supporting relationships. I know this from experience. Keeping one's focus is especially difficult in times of stress (which is often), or when one is discouraged (which for some people, can also be often). To help a Citizen Advocacy staff person keep her focus, someone in the organization — generally the board — must keep the coordinator's "feet to the fire," but in the context of a trusting, encouraging, helpful board-staff relationship. The function and responsibilities of a Citizen Advocacy coordinator must be clearly stated through policies, job descriptions, and most important, expectations. Clarity of staff function enables the coordinator to "be who she is, and do what she does," as a Citizen Advocacy coordinator whose primary function is to make matches and support relationships.

Also, there are innumerable activities that may be worth doing, but are not Citizen Advocacy. The staff of a Citizen Advocacy program does not engage in other forms of advocacy, public education, or become advocates themselves. Should they become advocates in their capacity as coordinators, they would be paid professional advocates, not voluntary citizen advocates. A Citizen Advocacy coordinator must focus on finding advocates for a wide range of devalued people. Should the coordinator become a personal advocate for people rather than recruiting advocates for them, the coordinator will quickly become preoccupied and probably overwhelmed, which will distract her from facilitating Citizen Advocacy. Finally, when Citizen Advocacy staff become advocates as part of their paid role, they perpetuate the stereotype that only paid professionals will become involved in the lives of devalued people, which undermines the very concept of Citizen Advocacy.

This is not to say that Citizen Advocacy coordinators should not be personally engaged in the life of someone with a disability. Of course they should — but on their own time. The benefits of personal engagement apply to Citizen Advocacy coordinators because they too, are people, and when they are not being coordinators, they are citizens. However, a Citizen Advocacy coordinator must be careful not to confuse people (including the protégé) as to when he or she is acting as a private citizen and when as a Citizen Advocacy coordinator.

Clarity of staff function is also relevant to what citizen advocates can expect from the Citizen Advocacy office. The role of the coordinator is to support, not supplant, Citizen Advocacy relationships. Sometimes Citizen Advocacy coordinators end up "taking over" the citizen advocate's role with good intentions. For example, if a coordinator goes with an advocate to a human service planning meeting with the intention of supporting the advocate, the perception by service-providing agencies may be that the "advocate-in-charge has brought along her volunteer to our inter-disciplinary meeting." This perception will disempower the advocate's role, and provide a handy target for the wrath of the agencies involved should the advocacy become adversarial. In the long run, citizens have more power than professionals, because their motivation for advocacy is a genuine, freely-given and freely-chosen relationship based on unconflicted concern for the protégé.

Diversity of Relationships

A Citizen Advocacy program recruits advocates for people

who have a wide range of identities and needs, and so citizen advocates fill a wide range of flexible roles.

Given the diversity of human beings, devalued people have a wide variety of identities, interests, needs and vulnerabilities. Most Citizen Advocacy programs recruit advocates for people of all ages, including the very young and the very old. Individual programs may focus on certain types of disabilities, but the people they find advocates for may still have a wide range of impairments. Some Citizen Advocacy programs give particular priority to people with significant impairments, since such people tend to be more vulnerable. However, many people with even minor impairments may need a strong ally or spokesperson to defend their interests.

Citizen Advocacy programs learn about people with disabilities who live in a variety of settings, including nursing homes, boarding homes, private homes, group homes, institutions, jails, and on the street. The people with disabilities for whom they find advocates are also involved in a variety of human service programs: sheltered workshops, day-activity programs, mental health outpatient centers, segregated schools, employment training programs, and other programs. Some people with disabilities — though unfortunately, relatively few — are in neighborhood schools or regular employment.

Citizen Advocacy is therefore not limited to any single role, such as only friends, or only spokespersons, but includes many flexible role options according to the unique identity of each person who needs an advocate. Some relationships center on basic needs for friendship, support and love. Other relationships are more involved with solving practical problems. Many, perhaps most, relationships involve both emotional and practical dimensions. A citizen advocate might be a roommate, adoptive parent, guardian, sponsor, mentor, advisor, ally, protector, good neighbor, and/or friend. Some examples of initial roles for a citizen advocate include:

Advocate Spokesperson
An advocate who vigorously represents the interest of a devalued person in situations in which that person's rights are, or are at risk

of, being compromised.

Advocate Guide
An advocate who assists with practical problem-solving such as housing, budgeting, shopping, transportation, etc.

Guardian
An advocate who assumes court-appointed responsibility for making important decisions for a person who is unable to make such decisions.

Representative Payee
An advocate who manages and oversees the finances for someone who cannot manage his own money. Typically a representative payee receives the monthly disability payment or other benefit and ensures that the funds are used appropriately according to individual needs and circumstances.

Advocate Monitor
An advocate who monitors and reviews services being provided to his protégé, and holds the service provider accountable for the quality of those services.

Adoptive Parent
An advocate who assumes the legal parental responsibility and moral obligations for a child as a member of his own family.

Friend
An advocate who has genuine affection for his protégé and shares of himself or herself in a mutual relationship.

Co-Advocate
An advocate who shares his advocacy on behalf of a protégé with another advocate, although usually in different roles.

Financial Supporter
An advocate who provides funds to assist someone with a disabili-

ty in financial crisis or for specific material needs.

Crisis Advocate
An advocate who responds to someone in a crisis or emergency situation and works to resolve a specific problem or crisis.

Legal Assistance Advocate
An attorney willing to give occasional *pro bono* legal assistance to a person with a disability.

Life-sharer
An advocate who invites his protégé to share his home.

Mentor
An advocate who assumes a role of a trusted teacher and takes a personal interest in advancing the personal and professional growth of her protégé.

Other Roles
Citizen advocates may assume any number of roles, according to the needs, interests, and capacities of the advocate and protégé, such as advisor, partner, fellow club member, protector, ally and so on.

In practice, citizen advocates often assume more than one role, and may have different roles in a person's life at different times. Like all human relationships, Citizen Advocacy relationships entail different degrees of demand. Some relationships can be intense, with a high degree of daily involvement, such as adoption. Other relationships call for more moderate degrees of involvement, and some relationships may only involve occasional support.

When Citizen Advocacy was first conceived, the principle of diversity was intended as a social change strategy, and not necessarily as a defining principle of Citizen Advocacy. As a strategy for social change, the diversity principle enables Citizen Advocacy programs to become more firmly rooted in the fabric of community life. However, a Citizen Advocacy program could, for legitimate purposes, decide to focus on finding citizen advocates for a narrower range of people and still be Citizen Advocacy. For example, a Citizen Advocacy program could be designed specifically for children with AIDS, or for homeless people, or for any devalued group. Arranging matches for such people could incorporate the principles of Citizen Advocacy and thus be a bona fide Citizen Advocacy program. To my knowledge, this kind of Citizen Advocacy program does not yet exist, but designing such a program is an interesting possibility.

Positive Interpretations of Devalued People (Imagery)

Citizen Advocacy strives to counter the negative images so commonly associated with devalued people by promoting positive, dignifying images in whatever ways possible.

Images shape and influence how we perceive people. One of the reasons images are so powerful is that they convey messages without words. An image can impress a message upon a person's mind without the person even being aware of it. This is especially true when images are presented over and over again, and when there is a consistent theme to the messages conveyed. Advertisers are well aware of this fact, hence the billions of dollars spent annually on advertising.

Devalued people tend to be surrounded by negative images. Physical settings, personal appearance, language, activities, and written media all present images that contain symbolic meaning. Our society "brands" devalued people as different in a negative way through countless demeaning and usually false symbolic messages, many of which are found in human services. For example, a homeless shelter or nursing home may be located at the edge of town, or out of town, conveying the image that the people there do not really belong in the community. By congregating devalued people in segregated groupings, the message is that such people "belong with their own kind." Adolescents in a segregated school may color with crayons and engage in other childish activities year after year, which reinforces the perception that they are children who will never grow up. Fundraising efforts to support human service programs often appeal to charity and pity rather than enhancing the dignity of the people they serve. Child-like decorations commonly seen in nursing homes suggest that elderly people are in their second childhood. Shabby programs operated in run-down facilities portray people as worthless and trivial.

In other words, the company you keep, the things that you do, where and how you spend your time, how you speak (and how people speak about you), and your personal appearance influence what people think about you — and perhaps what you think about yourself.[31] Devalued people cannot afford to have negative messages sent out that deepen their devaluation. This kind of "advertising" confirms negative assumptions and stereotypes.

To reverse or at least not add to this, Citizen Advocacy tries to draw upon positive images, by using respectful, dignifying language, engaging in age-appropriate, value-conferring activities, and doing whatever it can to present people in a positive light. Citizen Advocacy programs strive to portray people with disabilities as human beings who have inherent dignity, deserve respect, and whose lives are every bit as important and valuable as anyone else's.

A Citizen Advocacy program should therefore be a model of positive interpretation of devalued people through all the messages it conveys via its office setting and location, the personal identity of the board and staff, the funding sources, the media and materials used, the sponsored activities, and any other images presented in carrying out its work.

The guiding principles of Citizen Advocacy help a Citizen Advocacy program be what it is and do what it does. That is, the principles of Citizen Advocacy define the identity of Citizen Advocacy. In other human endeavors, such as in the areas of law and politics, a lawyer incorporates legal principles in her practice;

---

[31] For further elaboration of imagery issues, see Wolfensberger W., and Thomas, S. (1983). *PASSING (Program Analysis of Service Systems' Implementation of Normalization Goals): Normalization criteria and ratings manual.* (2nd. ed.). Toronto: National Institute on Mental Retardation.

political parties define themselves by "platforms" or statements of principle that guide who they are and what they do. Likewise, Citizen Advocacy programs — if they profess to be Citizen Advocacy — need to live by their principles.

There are many worthwhile things to do in the world, including other legitimate forms of advocacy. Organizations that engage in a different form of advocacy, and which do not subscribe to the defining principles of Citizen Advocacy, should in all honesty define themselves as whatever they are, rather than call themselves Citizen Advocacy but do something different.

Careful implementation of the Citizen Advocacy principles calls for clear thinking and creative work. In this sense, the Citizen Advocacy principles enable thoughtful people to accomplish the mission and purpose of Citizen Advocacy with clarity and excellence. In addition to the Citizen Advocacy principles, there are other concepts that can be helpful to citizen advocates: avoiding social overprotection, emphasizing lasting relationships, and promoting adoption and other formal roles.

Avoiding Social Overprotection

People who have substantial physical or mental impairments almost always need a certain amount of support and protection, but they do need not to be "smothered" by overprotection. Most learning involves new challenges, and there is a certain dignity in being able to take reasonable risks from which a person can learn and grow. Giving enough, but not too much, help is a delicate balance.

Striking a balance between under-protection and over-protection depends on how dependent or independent a person is, or can be. In my early years of trying to have a positive impact in the lives of people with disabilities, the creed was "to make people independent." Those of us who worked in the deinstitutionalization era succeeded in making many people independent, but all too often, alone. Independence can be a lonely place. The loneliness and isolation we created in people's lives was a reflection of our mistaken belief that self-fulfillment is found in becoming independent, free, autonomous individuals. We became full of ourselves, disconnected from one another, and alone in our self-created cells of personal isolation, which we imposed on the very people who needed our help. This kind of independence separates, isolates and divides.

The credo of independence has given helping a bad name. In our foolish quest for self-reliance, we miss valuable opportunities to learn the lessons of relying on one another. The presence of human impairment, then, is an opportunity for vulnerable, imperfect human beings to "help each other be strong," as Louisa and Teresa taught us. Mutual engagement in one another's lives, in real and practical ways, gives meaning to our lives.

Of course, advocates need to be discerning about how much control or influence may be needed to protect a person's interests while supporting the level of autonomy of which that person is capable. Advocates should be particularly careful about assuming a formal role in a person's life (such as guardianship) in ways that unnecessarily infringe upon that person's liberties and autonomy. But, liberty and autonomy are not the highest good. A person who makes decisions that are clearly dangerous or harmful to his life needs someone to step in and protect him from his own actions.

Citizen Advocacy has been criticized by some people as "patronizing" or as maintaining a dependent role for people with disabilities. Such critics argue that asking someone to protect and defend the interests of a person with a disability does not promote empowerment and independence. In the extreme, some argue that no one has the prerogative to speak for another person.

In response to these criticisms, I would ask: who of us does not need the support of people around us? Who of us has not benefited from a strong voice raised on our behalf at some point in our lives? Is it not true that people with disabilities tend to be isolated? Doesn't a physical or mental impairment mean that some kind of support is usually needed to function in daily life? Some people, such as persons described as being in a coma or in a "persistent vegetative state," need a great deal of support just to stay alive. The amount of support a person needs in no way diminishes that person's dignity. Equality of value means equal dignity and equal worth as human beings, but it does not mean that everyone has equal ability, talent or capacities. Indeed, some people need support in order to express whatever autonomy they may be capable of exercising.

If we accept the notion that no one person should speak for another, then wounded, isolated and dependent people will be denied the support and assistance they need from fellow citizens. In a culture that represses vulnerability, we have our collective heads in the sand about just how vulnerable we are as human beings. In our individualistic pride, we strive towards self-reliance and illusory radical independence that isolate and separate us from one another. Striving to create and support interdependence with responsible human autonomy leads to a safer place, and to a more fulfilled life.

The Need for Lasting Relationships

Like anyone else, people who have been socially devalued need other people who will make substantive personal commitments to them. Some may need a certain amount of help and support for a specific reason and for a limited period of time, but most people need relationships that will last. This may be the case even when such a person may not need much practical help, but still needs friendship. As relationships grow and mature, many citizen advocates find themselves gladly engaged in lasting relationships, and would consider it unthinkable to break off the relationship. As with any genuine relationship, these bonds are open-ended and may last a lifetime.

Adoption and Other Formal Relationships

Citizen Advocacy programs on occasion support the adoption of children with disabilities who need a family. A family making a life-time commitment to a child or adolescent is perhaps the highest form of advocacy. Offering a child a family is life-giving for the family, and may be life-saving for the child.

Sometimes a sanction from a legally recognized authority is necessary for an advocate to have a standing in a person's life when a person is unable to make his own decisions. Therefore, other formal relationships, such as guardianship, representative payee, or power-of-attorney may be needed for specific reasons. This is often the case when such decisions involve a person's health, such as a medical proxy, or their finances, such as a trustee, or for other major life decisions.

A P P E N D I X B

Where to Find Information About
Citizen Advocacy

Citizen Advocacy has been in existence since 1970, and as of this writing, there are over 100 Citizen Advocacy programs around the world, including in the United States, Canada, the United Kingdom, and Australia. These programs vary in adherence to Citizen Advocacy principles, staffing and structure, numbers of matches, and sources of funding. A few states or provinces have statewide or provincial support offices, whose responsibilities include the fostering and development of local Citizen Advocacy programs in their respective state or province. State and provincial offices include:

United States
Georgia Advocacy Office, Inc.
100 Crescent Center, Suite 520
Tucker, Georgia 30084 USA
Phone: (404) 885-1234
Fax: (770) 414-2948
E-mail: info@thegao.org

Nebraska Advocacy Services
215 Centennial Mall South, Suite 522
Lincoln, Nebraska 68508 USA
Phone: (402) 474-3183
Fax: (402) 474-3274
E-mail: John@NAS-PA.org

Massachusetts Citizen Advocacy
P.O. Box 362
Orange, MA 01364 USA
Phone: (978) 249-7769
Fax: (413) 529-2567
E-mail: tpdoody@excite.com

Pennsylvania Citizen Advocacy
222 Quail Court
Baden, PA 15005
Phone: (724) 772-7497
Fax: (724) 772-8267
E-mail: guycaruso@aol.com

Wisconsin Coalition for Advocacy
16 North Carroll St., Suite 400
Madison, WI 53703 USA
Phone: (608) 267-0214
Fax: (608) 267-0368
E-mail: wcamsn@w-c-a.org

United Kingdom
Citizen Advocacy Information and Training
162 Lee Valley Technopark
Ashley Road
Tottenhamhale, London
UNITED KINGDOM
Phone: (02 08) 880-4545
Fax: 020-880-4113 (mark f.a.o. CAIT)
E-mail: cait@teleregion.co.uk

Australia

An informal network of Citizen Advocacy programmes in Australia has established a website that lists the various offices throughout the country, as well as individual contact information. The website address is: www.uow.edu.au/arts/sts/bmartin/CAN

For further information on the Citizen Advocacy Network in Australia, you can contact: brian_martin@uow.edu.AU

———

Perhaps the single most unifying activity of the Citizen Advocacy movement is the practice of external evaluation using the Citizen Advocacy Program Evaluation (CAPE) instrument. CAPE evaluations entail an intensive review whereby a team of people provides a comprehensive analysis and feedback for a local Citizen Advocacy program. The process generally takes four or five days, and includes interviews with advocates, people who have advocates, program staff, board members, funders, and supporters. The CAPE team uses an objective set of standards to evaluate the program's consistency (or inconsistency) with established Citizen Advocacy principles and sound practice (see Appendix A). CAPE evaluations not only provide useful (and sometimes crucial) guidance to a Citizen Advocacy program, but they also provide a forum for development and training for those who participate on the evaluation team.

A less frequent but important aspect of the Citizen Advocacy movement are conferences on state, regional, national, or international levels. These conferences provide valuable opportunities for the development of ties and relationships within the Citizen Advocacy movement. Another unifying feature of the Citizen Advocacy movement is that Citizen Advocacy programs generally show warm hospitality to people who are interested in learning about the day-to-day functions of Citizen Advocacy. Spending time with experienced Citizen Advocacy program coordinators and boards, and most importantly, meeting advocates and protégés, are the best ways to learn what Citizen Advocacy is all about. The Citizen Advocacy programs that permitted me to interview advocates in their program are examples of programs that are willing to share what they have learned. They are:

Chatham-Savannah Citizen Advocacy
127 Abercorn Street
Savannah, Georgia 41401 USA
Phone: (912) 236-5798
Fax: (912) 236-1028
E-mail: csca@savannahga.net

Grand Island Citizen Advocacy
1407 Newcastle Road, Suite #107
Grand Island, Nebraska 68801 USA
Phone: (308) 385-5542
Fax: (308) 385-5542
E-mail: ginecitizenadv@juno.com

Illawarra Citizen Advocacy
Suite 8, 128-134 Crown Street
P.O. Box 5134
Wollongong, New South Wales 2500
AUSTRALIA
Phone: 4229 4064
Fax: 4228 0406
E-mail: illawarraca@bigpond.com

One to One: Citizen Advocacy
650 Corporation Street, Suite 302
Beaver, Pennsylvania 15009 USA
Phone: (724) 775-4121
Fax: (724) 775-4188
E-mail: onetoone@timesnet.net

Springfield Citizen Advocacy
One Armory Square
Springfield, Massachusetts 01101 USA
Phone: (413) 737-7540
E-mail: springfieldcitizenadvocacy@yahoo.com

Winnipeg Citizen Advocacy
120 Maryland Street
Winnipeg, Manitoba R3G-1L
CANADA
Phone: (204) 783-6516
E-mail: wpgca@mts.net

Another resource is the CITIZEN ADVOCACY FORUM, of which I served as editor for 12 years. The FORUM is an international Citizen Advocacy journal that publishes articles, stories and position papers on any number of topics in Citizen Advocacy. Back issues of the FORUM may be purchased from One to One: Citizen Advocacy by contacting One to One at the address listed above. The CITIZEN ADVOCACY FORUM continues under the able guidance of Jennifer Cullen in Pennsylvania, assisted by Mitchel Peters in Western Australia. Readers are encouraged to submit articles for possible publication, and to subscribe to the Forum by contacting:

Jennifer Cullen, Editor
Citizen Advocacy Forum
209 Leewood Drive
Lower Burrell, Pennsylvania 15065 USA
Phone: (724) 226-9641
E-mail: jennifercullen@yahoo.com

Mitchel Peters, Associate Editor
52 Giuralt Road
Marangaroo, WA 6064
Australia
Phone: 08 9342 3778
E-mail: mpeters@primus.com.au

The Training Institute for Human Service Planning, Leadership and Change Agentry at Syracuse University, directed by Wolf Wolfensberger, Ph.D., provides workshops on social advocacy and related topics relevant to Citizen Advocacy. For a schedule of events, contact:

Training Coordinator
Training Institute for Human Service Planning, Leadership and Change Agentry
805 South Wilbur Ave., Ste. 3B1
Syracuse, New York 13204 USA
Phone: (315) 473-2978
Fax: (315) 473-2963

The Social Role Valorization Implementation Project (SRVIP) offers a number of workshops relevant to Citizen Advocacy, including topics related to the vulnerability of devalued people, especially in health care settings. They may be contacted at:

SRVIP
74 Elm St.
Worcester, MA 01609
(508) 752-3670
E-mail: SRVIP@mac.com

Additional information on social role valorization (SRV) and related workshops may be found on the SRV website: www.socialrolevalorization.com

The author may be contacted at:

Adam J. Hildebrand
10 C Street
Beaver, PA 15009
(508) 789-9540
E-mail: AdamJHildebrand@yahoo.com

ABOUT THE AUTHOR

ADAM (A.J.) HILDEBRAND was a founding member of One to One: Citizen Advocacy in Beaver, Pennsylvania, where he worked for 16 years as a Citizen Advocacy Coordinator. He is the past editor of the CITIZEN ADVOCACY FORUM, an international journal of the Citizen Advocacy movement. Mr. Hildebrand has been an associate of the Training Institute for Human Services Planning, Leadership, and Change Agentry directed by Wolf Wolfensberger, Ph.D. for many years, and he has consulted with many Citizen Advocacy and other advocacy organizations throughout the United States, Australia, and Canada. He is a doctoral candidate at Duquesne University in Pittsburgh in health care ethics, where he is specifically focusing on the heightened vulnerability of people with disabilities in health care settings. He is currently a consultant for Shriver Clinical Services in Massachusetts, an organization that serves people with disabilities who have complex medical needs.